Being Sick Sucks:

The Autoimmune Abyss

By

Emily A. Filmoᵣ

Table of Contents

Dedication

To Mom C,

I love you and will miss you forever

Inscription

Abyss [*uh*-**bis**]

noun

1. a deep, immeasurable space, gulf, or cavity; vast chasm.
2. anything that seems to be without end or is impossible to
    measure, define, or comprehend...[1]

"... for when you gaze long into the abyss.

The abyss gazes also into you."

Friedrich W. Nietzsche[2]

"Embrace the void and have the courage to exist."

Daniel Howell[3]

Content Warnings

I cuss. I make crude jokes. I am honest about the fucking harsh realities of living with chronic, sometimes uncontrolled, illness. I talk in depth about suicidal ideation in Chapter 4. I talk about racism, homophobia, transphobia, religious abuse, medical abuse, depression, anxiety, body image issues, bodily functions, and more throughout the book.

If you aren't ready for these topics and how they fuck with people living with chronic illness you are not ready for me.

Prologue

"It is a beautiful day, and it is great to be alive!"

The Hon. Jakob Th. Möller, Iceland

You may wonder why I am quoting a judge. The Hon. Möller is a Former Judge at the International Human Rights Chamber for Bosnia and Herzegovina. He is a Former Chief of the Communications Branch of the Office of the High Commissioner of Human Rights at the *United Nations* (OHCHR). He is a current Board Advisor at a Non-Governmental Organization called, The Centre for Civil and Political Rights (CCPR Centre).[4] I met him as one of my professors of Human Rights at the University of Tulsa's Human Rights Institute in Geneve, Switzerland, in 2003.

The Hon. Möller started each morning of our class with the quote above in a beautiful, whimsical voice. If a judge adjudicating some of the worst crimes against humanity can continue to choose to start each morning with this as his attitude, I've always felt it was my responsibility to do so as well. This partially inspired my *Beautiful Day* children's books, and also has encouraged my continuing to seek out music for solace when faced with difficulties.

PLAYLIST AND SONG RECOMMENDATIONS are included in the chapter headings.

Music is intertwined with all my life's experiences. My good childhood memories are filled with relatives draped around my grandparents' dining room table, doo-wopping, folk singing, and hymning all the old church songs for hours until, eventually, each of us kids dropped off and our snores drowned them out from the next room. My Grammy hummed her way through over ninety years of life, five kids, thirteen grandkids, and so many hours of "piddling around" through her house. On the good days, we sang showtunes in the car on the way to school, the store, or to go look at the leaves. I was in musicals, tried to learn instruments, and even briefly took voice lessons in college right before I got sick.

I still try to sing every day, sometimes on-key and sometimes not. Sometimes quietly, sometimes loud. It depends on my energy and my voice. I, at least, listen to music every day. I "dance," in small movements, while I cook, in my seat at the rink, while I homeschooled Sage, and always in the car. I may have secretly made chair dancing cool, even if "So You Think You Can Dance" doesn't know it. There isn't a moment in which I can't find a song...good or bad.

My best friend, Jaime, taught me that singing made up songs or inserting your own name and life into a preexisting song (try it — it is fun!) can brighten any shitty day. This is a motto to live by which I highly recommend! My favorite show, by the way, does this. One of Marshall's schticks on *How I Met Your Mother* is to make up ridiculous songs about himself. They are nearly always funny, but often mundane. Sometimes the songs are self-deprecating. Mostly he just describes what he is doing. It is *legend*-wait-for-it-*dary*. Legendary! In any event, they are a way to blow out some inner angst and a part of Marshall's whole character building; he is one of the most authentic, happiest, loveliest, and yet flawed characters ever to grace the airwaves. I always thought it was because they made him so real and approachable.

Finally, Scott and I have instilled a love of the arts, played music, and shared the presence and power of music in history in our home. We have tried to emphasize that music can encapsulate so much for a moment. It holds emotions, unlocks pent up fears, and motivates people. Music helps grieve, gives release, makes one laugh, and brings joy. Music helps implant memories, good and bad.

I enjoy a neurological gift called *synesthesia*.[5] I didn't know it was a difference for most of my life. I thought everyone saw the world in 3-D like this! Before I explain, let me assure you, it is not hallucinating, it is some type of connection or crossing of senses (two or more at a time). My understanding is that it is not uncommon to see it in people who have other sensory sensitivities, which I do (I can't wear rough shirts, strong noxious smells bother me and get "stuck" in my nose, sometimes for more than a day after I am no longer near that smell, loud noises make my eyes hurt, etc.).

Here are a couple of examples of my beautiful associations thanks to synesthesia. When I hear music, I see colors dancing along to the notes. When I think about colors, they have personalities, and some have strong smells (mostly pleasant). When I think about letters and numbers, they have beautiful colors. For instance, "B" is bright royal blue, but "b" is light sky blue. "H" is bright orange and "h" is peachy pink or almost light salmon. The number "1" is lipstick red and the number "3" is canary yellow. Letters and numbers also have genders. When I was a kid, I made up whole plays in my head using the characters of letters and numbers! In other words, the world is very beautiful, rich, and stimulating.

The reason I explain synesthesia is to help you understand what the playlist and the individual songs listed with each chapter have to do with the book. In many cases, I had a song playing in my head as I wrote a chapter. In some cases, when I went back to re-read a chapter a song struck me as "the" song for the chapter. Sometimes, I knew there was a song that I could "feel" but had to search online, and then when I found it, I knew! It is really like I have a symphony and a colorful cartoon always playing in the background of my life.

No matter how I came up with the song, each chapter title is accompanied by a song that touches me, somehow, pertaining to that specific topic. It reminds me of the background to a movie, how there is nearly always music playing behind a scene that helps set the mood and/or echoes the scene.

If you are moved to do so, I encourage you to take a quick break to listen to the songs before or with each chapter or listen to them all after you've read the book. I have made a playlist to assist you in finding the songs and have also included some other songs that didn't fit the chapters exactly but echoes my mood while writing the book! I could probably find a thousand pertinent songs to include in the playlist, but just like writing a book, you must find somewhere to cut yourself off.

For reference, I started the book in mid-November 2022, finished the first draft on February 28, 2023 (in a synchronistic turn of the universe, on Rare Disease Day). I put the book away for a few months and am back to do a final edit in mid-November 2023. Because of the ever-changing, circular nature but also universality of this disease, I have decided to edit details lightly. If there is a major change to my health in November 2023, that I feel you need to know within a particular chapter that I cannot easily edit, I will add it in parentheses. I realize now, all these months later, if I keep waiting for a "resolution" or to get better...I will never get this book out.

I've included links to the playlists on Apple and YouTube; the songs that are specifically mentioned in the book are listed in order, with other songs included after that have some meaning o me relatated to the book. You should also be able to find them by search for my name and the playlist name, "Being Sick Sucks;" or just play the songs individually. Please feel free to listen to any or all in any order. They are suggestions!

Apple Playlist: https://music.apple.com/us/playlist/being-sick-sucks/pl.u-55D6XW5FV6PLDk

YouTube Playlist: https://youtube.com/playlist?list=PLpX4K61rd-3_mwK6OUm2-B5QhS9KC6H7_

I hope you will find a way to make music or poetry or art or books or gazing at nature or anything else that helps you feel connection a part of your daily life because if you are living with chronic illness or mental illness or sadness or any of a myriad of other things that ail the human race, because even though I am taking the time in this book to sludge through the drudgery of being sick, we need things to remind us that "It is [indeed] a beautiful day and it is great to be alive!"

Enjoy the playlist and take care of yourself!

Love,

Emily

Before you start the book, listen to *"Blackbird," by The Beatles* and *"Moments," by Hollow Coves.*

Chapter 1
Why Being Sick Sucks

———

"The Story," by Sara Ramirez,

originally by Brandi Carlile

Life is full of influential people and pivotal moments. I'm not talking about the people on the news. I'm not talking about politicians. They don't know anything about your life or my life. I am talking about a life-long friend, friend in a support group, a neighbor, the person who cuts your lawn, the person who checks you out at the grocery store; it can be your doctor, your therapist, or your childhood teacher. It can also be your friend, your child, your spouse, or a stranger on the street...if only you can hear them speak.

A life-changing moment can be big or small. It can be a walk in the park or a move across the country. It can be changing jobs or can be a hearing in front of a disability judge. It can even be a simple dinner conversation on a night at home with your family. *All* these people, all these moments, can affect you. Any one of these can suddenly give you some piece of advice, a piece of information you didn't have before, a moment of divinity, clarity, or bliss...things that can help you live a better life, to transform your experience into something marvelous despite disease and to know *who you are* regardless of what is happening *within* your body...

...but yeah, if you came here for help finding that, this time, this isn't your fucking book.

This book is about the shit. The bad stuff. The things that happen to people with autoimmune disease when no one else is paying attention. This is my follow-up to *The Marvelous Transformation: Living Well with Autoimmune Disease*[6] (TMT) in which I explored how I've managed to have a happy life despite being ill.

However, I want to be very clear that this is not an extension of *The Marvelous Transformation*; it is almost its inverse. While still being written with the intent to help you, I want to enlighten you, lighten your load, maybe even to entertain while shedding light on the BS of autoimmune disease.

The problem with, or maybe the beauty of, the passage of time, is that I am not the same person, today, as I was when I wrote TMT. I am irrecoverably changed by my illness, and I don't think this is always for the better. I do not always try to find the "bright side." I do not always try to find the positive way out of my negative thoughts, and I certainly do not hide from the dark thoughts and feelings that accompany chronic illness. This book is the flip side of the TMT coin. It will expose the BS because *being sick sucks*.

However, I am also still the same in other ways. I am still loyal. I am still loving. I still expend too much energy doing the things that are dangerous to my body because parts of me are in denial of how sick I am.

...and...I am still funny — unless you ask my kids. Or at least I can still find "gallows humor" in horrible situations. I can't turn that off, even in the worst of times I crack jokes for release. I hope you find those jokes to be a sort of release as well, because, well, if we can't laugh at the horrible then the only thing left to do is cry.

I wrote TMT over eight years ago and life looks a lot different now. I have an even harder time with meds. My body is older and sicker. I have more diagnoses.

And I still live much of my life in my self-directed, *chosen*, bliss. I still have a beautiful family. I have support. I have amazing friends. I still have love.

So much love that I think sometimes *there has been a cosmic mistake.*

I worry I will wake up and it will all be gone; that I don't deserve this much love! That I got too much and others need it more. My medications that keep me kicking can also play tricks on my mind to turn me into a raving bitch (Sorry, Scott). They can also make my brain question the worth of my existence.

What an oxymoron to have medication-induced thoughts that I shouldn't be alive anymore or that my care, the cost of my care, and the burden of taking care of me has become too much for my husband when I have fought so hard to be here. I *am* fighting so hard to be here. The thought that my brain is betraying me as much as my body is; well, *that* is almost unbearable.

Ironically, I don't know many people who love being alive like I do. It's annoying, really...to me as much as to others!

I literally stop to smell flowers. I hug trees. I love to lie down in the grass and watch the clouds (as long as someone is there to help me up). I can sit for hours to watch the wind brush over a lake. Cattails and reeds waving in marshes as the wind tickles them bring me such peace and joy.

The northern Hoarfrost[7] startled me the first time I saw it. I wondered if I was imagining it because its majesty is unmatched. Since moving to Minnesota, it's like I've been transported to Alice's *Wonderland* because it seems impossible to find so much beauty and nature so close to home. It's not just winter, although I have a newfound appreciation for the cold and pristine soundless snowy months. I stop to take photos of a lone flower poking through a sidewalk because of the brilliance in its impossibility and tenacity. The colors of the sky seem to fascinate me far more than others.

I love my people so fiercely I sometimes overwhelm them (ahem, teenagers grow out of that, right?). I "dance" in my seat when I watch my daughter's figure skating practice no matter how embarrassing (teenagers grow out of that too, right?). I sing as loud as my weakened voice will let me. I cook elaborate meals and try new things in the kitchen; yet I hate recipes. The richer, the more varied the food the better (within our allergies — how unfair to have a family of foodies befallen with multiple food allergies!). I cry and sob equally with happiness as I do with sadness and grief. I live with open arms and an open heart and would *never* willingly decide to end my life.

But my innermost thoughts are dark, especially when alone. I feel sometimes like I am floating in an infinite abyss, tethered and weighted only by pain, fear, and utter despair. I am alone — surrounded by my loves and hundreds of caring well-wishers, both in real life and online, but still, always completely alone in the actual internal experience of the agony of the mercilessness of this disease.

I have pumped my body full of medications, herbs, vitamins, and organic foods. I have dabbed on and smeared myself with lotions, creams, oils, tinctures, and everything else I can find. I've meditated, needled, vibrated, twisted, detoxed, and sweated my body in every imaginable way. I have listened to the doctors, healers, and anyone else who knows anything about autoimmune disease for any tidbit that could change my circumstance, including people who are guessing! I've investigated or chased every fucking unicorn fart and sparkly rainbow that has ever looked promising to stop the autoimmune terrorist gripping my body.

These remedies and medications may work for a minute, but eventually they stop, or I get some unknown, rare side effect. I've also stopped or reduced the things that increase inflammation or have increased symptoms in my body. I even gave up my big macs, sausage egg biscuits, biscuits and gravy, flour tortillas, and croissants, when we realized I had problems with gluten a dozen years ago for gods' sakes!

I try to keep a positive attitude as mentioned in TMT because all the current wisdom and peer-reviewed studies say doing so leads to the best outcomes when living with chronic illness, especially when working with new medications and chronic illness wellness overall. But sometimes I just scream, "I've had enough! **Just work** [meds], damnit! Leave me alone [DM]!"

In the eight ensuing years since writing TMT, I now have the perspective of someone who has lived with the disease for roughly twenty-eight years. That's eight more years of this tyrant ravaging my body. Eight more years of hosting the most unwelcome "guest" who will not leave. Eight more years of horrible, I mean helpful, chemicals coursing through my veins. Eight more years of side effects and failed treatments. Eight more years of damage, both physical and emotional. Eight more years of trying to smile my way through this unrelenting bullshit; but the truth is sometimes that smiling feels like a big-fat-fucking-lie.

In the fall of 2022, I made several Facebook posts detailing how bad my weakness/stamina, treatment side effects, skin ulcers, scalp plaques, digestion, migraines, fatigue, pain, frustration, and countless other symptoms were. I make these posts to educate and explain the disease, but also as a measure of support for my friends in the chronic illness community because so often we question ourselves. I question myself;

how can I have all of this continuing to go wrong even though I am on daily Medrol and was (at the time) three years into consistent home infusions of subcutaneous immunoglobulin (SCIG) treatments?

Look, I am grateful for my minimal muscular improvements. I can go for walks with Scott and Sage for more than 15-20 minutes, sometimes even an hour! I can dress myself most days without assistance — yea for me! I can walk up the stairs without (literally) pulling myself with my arms or crawling, as in the past. I haven't consistently used my cane or walker in a few years. Now I need some wood to knock on!

But I am foggy, uncoordinated, and clumsy. I cannot safely cut vegetables alone. I constantly drop things. When I cook, I drop the spoon or splatter hot grease on myself multiple times a day. I fall easily. I cannot take a shower or fold laundry without exhausting to the point of needing a nap or at least a 15 (or more) minute rest. Too much laundry folding, or even typing on this very computer, at once sets off muscle spasms and tightness that lasts for days and usually leads to a migraine.

I continue to be plagued with horrendous pain, continued weakness and deconditioning, the side effects of my SCIG, migraines, and so much more. And my skin, my poor, prematurely aging, withering skin. My rash feels like the constant sound of the heart beating in Edgar Allen Poe's "Tell-Tale Heart."[8] It never stops pulsating, itching, rumbling, burning, and vibrating underneath the surface. I sometimes get this searing pain I call "fire ants." It is enough to want to tear my eyes and ears out; and scratch through to see if there is something underneath that could be removed and end the infernal suffering. Please do not confuse this with any desire for self-harm, this is a feeling that something is living under my skin and torturing me twenty-four hours a day, burning me from the inside out.

AFTER NOTING THE DOWNWARD pattern of these posts, my sweet friend, Connie, asked me, "Why are you not telling this part: 'the dark side' of your current story?"

I laughed, "What on earth do you mean? Between posting the sweet sleeping pictures of my dog, River 'The Asshole' Filmore, pictures of the beautiful, tranquil nature of Minnesota's lakes (many of which have Scott and me grinning in the foreground — selfie time!), Sage's skating videos, Rickey's art, my posts advocating human rights peppered with political rants...I **am** telling this story! That's why I share all the 'TMI' after the TMT on Facebook! Because I figure it helps others know they aren't the only ones, and to see that even *I, 'the live happy with disease woman,'* have bad days. A lot of them lately...but..."

She chuckled and said, "Yeah, you are doing great at helping your friend list, but let's be honest, you don't have a far reach. Write it in a book. Get it out." We laughed and I said I'd think about it.

But honestly, being sick means finite energy. It means I didn't really market TMT very well (although when I did, I **loved** talking to people), and disappointing sales showed it. It means I won't be able to go out to market this book well which makes me doubt even writing it.

But, what the hell! **Being Sick Sucks**. So, here I am, let's try! I guess I'm going to tell "the dark side" (Hey there, Star Wars fans!) I'll tell you all the shit of my Autoimmune Abyss. The merry-go-round of symptoms. The awful experiences of medication allergies and adverse responses including the ones that made part of my brain momentarily suicidal (yes, twice), the doctor appointments from hell...all of it.

I'm going to share the darkest parts of my thoughts, even the ones that scare me, to de-taboo this shit. I want to demystify and expose some of the things I have gone through, continue to go through, because while it isn't the same for every person, the feedback I get from my chronic illness community is there are some common threads of experience, and sometimes just knowing that you aren't the only person who heard *that*, felt *that*, was treated like *that*, is helpful, is galvanizing, helps to take a little dignity and power back.

I will share some of the deepest ugliest parts of myself so you can know what you are experiencing is part of our "normal" and so you can be armed with some of my coping mechanisms, no scratch that, living mechanisms. I'm not talking about meditation. I still do that too, but that doesn't always work when you are in the ongoing, awful pit of despair. I guess I'll share how it feels to be stymied by the assholes at insurance companies and nurses who belittle me, ER docs who think they know me after seeing my med list but have never heard the word "dermatomyositis" in their lives and how I respond! I'm going to, as my daughter would say, *spill the tea* on this never-ending fucking abyss of autoimmune disease. I may give some hints on how to handle them along the way, but mostly, I think I just want to expose the shit.

By the way in case you didn't catch it, I cuss...a lot. It's who I am. I think there is an elegance and strength in using the right word at the right time, especially a cuss word. It won't stop after this introduction, so if you don't like cussing, this book may not be for you, but I'm also going to talk about jack ass doctors, explosive poop, blood, racism, homophobia, transphobia, religious abuse, and medical abuse, so if direct honesty about the literal and figurative shit of the world is offensive to you, then this may not be the book for you...because I am not going to pull any punches.

Besides, there was a study that showed that people who "swear" are more trustworthy and have high integrity,[9] soooo would you rather listen to someone who is polite but "hides the poop" or a woman who cusses like a sailor but tells the truth? I'm firmly on team "let it all out!"

I am a firm proponent of saying what you mean; and always, always, meaning what you say. I taught my kids to be brave enough to say what they mean and mean what they say. I also taught them to respect the sensitivities of the people around them, but if you say, "Oh snap!" with the same energy and anger behind it as "oh shit!" there is no difference. You are just trying to please a made-up societal standard. So, if the problem is with the phrase, "Oh shit!" maybe it is time to address the problem that led to the feeling behind it!

In other words, why are people with autoimmune disease continuing to suffer physically and being ignored inevitably, at one time or another, in every possible way, by the very people who should care the most (family), who should be helping them (doctors), by medications that are harming them (because the pharmaceutical companies do not disclose dangerous side effects), missing out on treatments (because insurance companies want to play games with our lives to save money or delay paying), while spending hours and hours fighting for their rights (on the phone with people who can't even pronounce their disease!)?

In fact, I recently made a comment to my daughter Sage that the hospital should be paying me for the number of calls I made over a specific bill (they can't get our address right ad keep saying they have fixed it but do not) and I think I should call our senator to suggest a law that patients get reimbursed for when providers or insurance cost them time (especially because sick patients should be taking care of ourselves not wasting time on phone queues fighting with them to fix our records, approve our meds, pay our bills, etc.). She answered, "Or here's a thought, how about we just get them to provide universal healthcare since it is a Universal Human Right and cut out the bullshit."

I was floored. I've spent so much time and energy in the past advocating, screaming, really, for Universal Healthcare, but when it was my turn and I was fighting to get my address changed for six months — they beat me down — I forgot my own belief system and felt defeated. (This isn't the first time, it happens when they deny a medication for my rare disease and I spend hour upon hour to get approval because a prostate specialist in some small town who has never heard of my disease denies my medication without even reading about dermatomyositis because he has denial quotas.) Anyway, I was so proud that she could remind me of the bigger picture. We deserve better than this abusive system where patients are treated like discarded candy wrappers.

But...I digress...

I'm doing this book because, as my lovely friend pointed out to me, my ideas, guidance, tools, and methods in *The Marvelous Transformation* work (and I've been told that they do over and over and over) but you must be ready to be uplifted and reminded of your magnificence. You must be ready to transcend the physical part of disease to embrace *who you really are*. And sometimes we just aren't there.

Take me. I wrote the damn book. I tried to read it.

I couldn't.

I wasn't ready for it.

I wasn't in a place to transcend shit.

The only high I was getting was from weed — and that was to get rid of some shooting nerve pain. In fact, I was reading a digital copy on my phone, but if it was a paperback, I would have thrown it across the room!

Sometimes, like that day[10], you just want to feel the muck. You want to give yourself permission to wallow. And, honestly, if you are not strong enough to give it to yourself, you want someone to tell you, "Hey, it's okay to wallow today and cry it out."

Well, here's your permission. I have a great support system around me that tells me, and so I am here to tell you today: *Let that shit out, baby.*

If you need to...You can stop pretending you believe things will be better if you meditate, or burn enough incense, or put on enough essential oils, or repeat enough mantras, or take enough vitamins, or tell enough jokes, or say enough prayers, or smile enough, or drink enough water, or walk enough miles, or do enough sun salutations, or look on the bright side enough, or say enough affirmations, or count enough blessings, or list enough moments of gratitude, or drink enough coffee, or run enough errands, or cook enough meals, or clean your house enough, or walk the dog, or take out the trash, or, or, or, or...sometimes you want to hear that someone else gets there too, and know it's okay to acknowledge the abyss we live in with autoimmune disease and say, "fuck it," feel it, acknowledge it, let it flow through you and out of you, and know that for today:

It is okay to not be okay.

Chapter 2
Who Am I?
Why Do You Care About What I Have to Say?

"You've Got a Friend in Me," by Randy Newman, from Toy Story

I'm really nobody. I'm just a patient who has lived this bullshit for over twenty-eight years.

My husband Scott and I have a supernatural love that I am pretty sure was part of the universe's original big bang. He's sweet and calm when I am not. That song by The Chicks, *Easy Silence*? It was written years before I met him; but when I met Scott, I knew what they meant. I am pretty sure that fate and all the stars used it to make sure I knew he was my person. It is true that he is much nicer, inside and out, than me. He is sweet, cute, and funny, but shy, and saves his humor and best million-watt smiles for me and our kids. He is a dedicated dad and husband and immensely hard-working. I'm pretty sure at one point of our life an entire group of neighbors didn't even believe he existed and that I had made him up because he worked so much.

Most notably, for our purposes here, he has always been a wonderful health partner and caretaker. He gives me my shots and home infusions even though as a tax and trust and estates wonk he doesn't have any interest in medicine. He figured prominently in TMT. I based the caregiver tips on how much he helps me. He does all these things and is a consistent emotional-support-giver on top of being my love... even when the increased doses of steroids alter the chemistry of my brain and make me say horrible, terrible, no-good, awful things... like the last time I increased my steroids significantly.

Ugh. Hmpf. Please, don't make me re-live those weeks and please don't ever let me be like that again.

Side note: Living through yet another bout of steroid induced rage makes me pretty sure that the witch in Hansel and Gretel was on steroids for two reasons. First, she was a stark, raving, angry, uncontrollable shrew for seemingly no good reason. Second, she was insatiably hungry and couldn't stop eating. I don't believe in Evil, but steroids...yep...they are evil if Evil exists. Yet, I can't get away from them. I try. Believe me. The lower doses seem to be tolerable, the higher ones, well, keep your candy house and sensitive feelings away from me!

We have two kids. Sage is almost eighteen and Rickey is thirty. Rick is thriving and living his artist's dream in LA with his fiancé Tiffany who is working in human rights. They are all smart, strong, creative, loving, impressively kindhearted, and they know who they are! Sometimes Scott and I sit back and wonder how these wonderful beings are "ours" but then we realize they aren't. It's the opposite. *We are theirs*. We are just stewards who helped them navigate finding themselves; and no matter what, we see them as perfection.

Scott, Sage, and I moved to Minnesota in 2021 to help Sage fulfill part of her figure skating ambitions of working with a high-level coach she loved, within a training program aligned with our ethics and beliefs of how to treat kids. It has been a dream come true. It also gave us a much needed, and appreciated, change of scenery! We are so happy we did it. It was the right thing for all of us, especially as Rick and Tiff moved to LA around the same time and it all worked out... plus, I still talk to my dad — nearly every day, whether he wants to or not! Poor guy! *wink wink*

When I got mono at college, I was virtually alone except for a few other 19-year-olds. My parents came to get me in a snowstorm. The doctor thought I had strep and had given me an antibiotic. It caused a reaction with the mono; making me blow up like a baboon holding an inflated balloon with the addition of a red bumpy rash. It did a ton of internal stuff, too. It is what was believed to take my over-sensitive body (plagued throughout childhood with recurrent infections, rashes, aches, pains, sun sensitivities, and undefined malaises) into full-blown autoimmune disease. I was home for a long, long month while the initial reaction calmed down...and mono worked its way out before I was allowed to go back to college.

It took 7-8 years to be finally diagnosed, but along the way I was mocked, minimized, misdiagnosed, and ignored by much of the medical establishment. (This was my first conscious experience with what I now consider to be medical abuse, however looking back my dad and I believe I was gaslighted my entire childhood when doctors told my parents I was over-sensitive and looking for attention when my lips blew up like pillows, kept getting heat stroke, or had intractable back pain.)

It wasn't until my rash became "defined" that a dermatologist did a biopsy and was able to deliver the word that would change my life: dermatomyositis.

He might as well had said, "dirty-martini-bloody-my-olive-itis" at that point because no one I asked had heard of it, including doctors, and in 2003 very few articles even existed (or at least came up when searching on the fairly sparse interwebs). What I did read scared the hell out of me. But I was also oddly, immensely relieved to know I had a diagnosis, a name to describe the hell I had been living.

I've detailed that long and arduous 7–8-year journey from onset to diagnosis to treatment in TMT. I went through many doctors and still, after being diagnosed, I was left without adequate treatment for a long time. Because of this thing ravaging my body, I had accumulated "sustained damage" — not only did I have current "active disease" but being sick so long without appropriate treatment had caused long-term damage.

The western conventional meds made me sick. I pursued alternatives. They helped, until they didn't.

I went on the merry-go-round of steroids, IVIG (immunoglobulin), cellcept, imuran, methotrexate, plaquenil, quinacrine, and back again. There are others we discussed and didn't try because of the number and magnitude of my side effects. I interspersed acupuncture, Chinese medicinal herbs, chiropractic care, and everything else we could muster to maintain some kind of balance.

I had gone to law school before being diagnosed and while I still had hope that I may get better, studying human rights and international and comparative law. After graduating, and passing the Bar Exam, it became clear I would not be practicing law in any traditional sense. I tried a solo practice, but even those time commitments including keeping up on my CLEs, on top of trying to be a mom were too much for my sick and over-reactive body.

After mourning that it was clear I couldn't practice law, I let go of my law license. I eventually decided to use my mind and writing skills in other ways. One was that I started to write children's books and write about spiritual parenting. A serendipitous conversation with Neale Donald Walsh, the best-selling author of many books including *Conversations with God*, who was, at the time, also my personal writing mentor and the concurrent co-author of one of my books, *Conversations with God for* Parents, led me to write TMT.

I begged Neale to help me understand how I could be so happy in my life, be applying the spiritual principles of positive thinking, and yet not be able to "cure" myself of this wretched terrorist trying to kill my body. He explained that I wasn't doing anything wrong, by transcending the emotional pain, I was *successfully living with* illness. By continuing to have a happy life I **was** beating dermatomyositis, just not in the ways in which we normally think.

This reframing was crucial, at the time, to both my mental and spiritual health as well as maybe helping to improve my physical wellbeing. He also encouraged me to share my story, to write TMT because he thought I could help others see the good, bad and the ugly of illness, and come out stronger and ready to face the disease more fully.

I wrote TMT and while I was too sick to market it as well as I, or my publisher, would have liked, the response from the people who read it was staggering. They felt heard, seen, and understood. I thought, "Even if that is all I accomplish as a writer, I am happy. I'm a good mom, I am loved by my family, I helped people with my story, I am a 'success.'"

My conversations leading up to TMT's publication led to me meeting Jerry Williams in 2014. He had started a Facebook group called Polymyowhat? and was ready to start a full-blown non-profit along with Sandy Block. I jumped in (gingerly...how truly "jumpy" can you be with a muscle and skin disease?) and soon became a co-founding director of Myositis Support and Understanding (MSU), a non-profit 501(c)(3) organization for people with all forms of myositis (idiopathic inflammatory myopathies). The all-volunteer organization helps people with myositis, by people touched by myositis. One of the great parts of being involved in an organization run by people with your disease is knowing that you can be honest about your limitations, because we all understood when we could and couldn't participate. I helped build MSU and volunteered for it for nearly eight years until I retired from it last year. I am so proud of all the things we did together while I was with MSU as well as how it continues to grow.

I have talked to hundreds, maybe, thousands of people across the world with myositis and other autoimmune diseases due to my books and in my roles with MSU. Through the years I served as volunteer, VP, board advisor, group leader, writer, and more. I have enjoyed speaking with people privately, personally, and as a leader of MSU's online support groups and zoom support sessions. I also spoke at The Myositis Association's Annual International Patient Conference about the value of telling your story. I was honored to speak, in my capacity as a parenting writer at Dr. Shefali's *EVOLVE* parenting summit, and I have spoken to small groups about both parenting and living with illness.

I am proud to be published in a major medical journal, <u>Rheumatology</u>, because of a pain study we did at MSU in which I was an architect and author of the questions and which the MSU medical advisors later analyzed and published to show the prevalence of pain for myositis patients, the first study of myositis patients of its kind.

In my personal life, I believe that I have an obligation and duty to stay informed as a citizen, so while my physical limitations keep me from being as civically and politically active as I would like, I have joined learning groups and taken online seminars to better myself on the topics of human rights, anti-racism, Diversity, Equity, and Inclusion, and other topics (the online availability of these seminars is especially helpful and inclusive when you can do it in your own time and comfortable at home due to illness). I am politically involved when I can with my physical limitations, and read voraciously about the plight of people with chronic illness.

Besides TMT I have written two children's books about connecting with your child through shared activities and co-authored two parenting books.[11] I have written countless articles on illness, on parenting, on spirituality, as well as the intersection of each for both MSU and other publications including The Mighty, Nurture Parenting, Medium, CWG Connect, and more than my medication-addled mind can remember. I've been interviewed for podcasts and articles, stood on stage next to famous authors, and sat with people as they cried about their pain.

I've helped other patients write letters to insurance companies, called state boards of insurance with patients to get them advocacy help, and just about any other quiet advocacy I could do within the confines of being stuck. Stuck with illness. Stuck with migraines. Stuck with a body who doesn't care that this is not the life I didn't fucking chose.

When the pandemic was first raging I did as much as I could to educate people about the aftereffects of a viral infection. While stuck at home and scared shitless of this unknown threat, I sewed hundreds of masks that I donated to group homes and individuals for free when masks were still impossible to find. When the vaccines were first available to the public and immune suppressed people with autoimmune disease were not clearly being prioritized, I advocated with the CDC, my state, and the American College of Rheumatology to have the wordage corrected.

I wake up most mornings and terrifyingly briefly I forget my body isn't really mine. I hear my brain ticking, I know my thoughts, I remember Who I Really Am inside, and then I try to move, and the pain, stiffness, swelling, and everything else comes crashing down. Other mornings I wake up in so much pain it is impossible to forget. Either way, every day, I grieve who I want to be, or who I thought I was, maybe even who I think I am for a foggy waking moment...every single fucking day. This isn't about acceptance. It's about that moment, in between when you are only your mind and you forget, and then the moment when you remember.

Yet, I am still the person my friends call to edit a letter or to pep them up before they make an important call, go on a job interview, or call to yell at, I mean argue with, their doctor or insurance company to get a medication covered, and I get great pleasure in doing those things because I am helping my friends. This helps me to remember that I am not worthless. It helps me through the times I feel like my purpose was stolen from me because sometimes I can't get past the feeling of knowing, wishing, and dying inside because I feel I was meant to be and do more than sit on the couch watching re-runs of *How I met Your Mother*.

I am writing this to make my life matter but also because if you are like I was when I tried to re-read TMT maybe you just need to hear from another person going through a similar experience that this shit is absolutely real. It sucks. It feels like a never-ending story, and the shit multiplies exponentially.

Maybe by hearing my story, told from this perspective, after TMT, when I couldn't meditate my own way out of a paper bag much less the pain and anguish of my DM, it will help you to know you aren't the only one. I, too, wrestle with that fear, that feeling every day, "Am I completely alone going through the weird the vicissitudes of this vile disease?"

Or, "Am I making it all up?" maybe all those asshole doctors at the beginning were right after all...

And I admit it.

I am worried that after all these years dermatomyositis is finally, slowly, taking *me* away from me.

I feel like I am losing myself.

That's it, that's my resume. I hope you will stick with me and see if I have something to offer you. If I can give voice to something you haven't been able to express before, or just to acknowledge something that you didn't know was "okay" to feel.

I recently read a poignant article on another topic that was pertinent to another part of my life. It struck a chord so deep inside me and gave words to feelings I have held so close but didn't know were true. After reading it I felt enlightened and lighter. It didn't change that situation, but it did make me feel *better* in some way.

I hope, even though I don't intend to offer you solutions here, you feel that same soul's recognition in reading this. I hope you will realize even though we probably haven't met that you've truly ...got *a friend in me...* and then maybe, someday, you and I will both be ready to read *The Marvelous Transformation*, and *Live Well with Autoimmune Disease*, together.

Chapter 3
Losing My "Religion," Twice

"Losing My Religion," by REM

My view of the world and universe has changed multiple times in the past three decades. I was born into and raised in the Catholic Church. For many reasons I left it in my twenties and went on a quest to find my own spirituality. I read holy texts and treatises from a multitude of the world's religions. I came to an understanding of myself and my place in the universe as a "new-age spiritual non-religious" person and that carried me for a couple of decades. Over the past few years, I have come to discard that mantle because I didn't appreciate how, in my opinion, it was twisted and misapplied. But I also decided I didn't want a label at all. I've decided labels are limiting when humans have the capacity to be limitless.

We found out a few years ago that I am partly, ethnically, Ashkenazi Jewish. I wasn't raised knowing this due to an indiscretion by my paternal grandmother that wasn't verified until we confirmed with a DNA test. As I said, we do not practice any religion, but I have extensively studied Jewish history for my entire adulthood, even before knowing my own roots. I am proud of my Jewish heritage, feel a strong desire to know and understand the plight of the Jewish Community and wish I knew my dad's biological family.

Now, if you were to ask me what I believe, my main belief is in Scott, Sage, Rickey, and Tiffany. They keep me going. They show me the real meaning of love. They *are* my definition of "love."

But beyond that, I guess there are a couple of words that loosely describe how I view the world.

Atheist:

Since it is the biggest and possibly most off-putting to many, I'll start here. I don't think there is a "person" who is a god. To most people, that makes me an atheist. Although, I think we are all divine, connected, and come from the same energy. I think we all have a part in whether we come together to make the human experience work or not.

I wish love (as in universal, agape love), empathy, and critical thinking were lauded as the most important skills to teach our children. We all can be "good" to each other, to give love to each other, and to find the "godliness" or greatness in each other but I do not think there is a person who is in charge or making decisions to punish and reward any of us; I think those ideas are all man-made mechanisms of control, which are failing, by the way. We would be better off teaching children to love one another because we are connected and every person is as important as every other person, not because some white-haired dude in the sky might smite them...

This would translate into a lot less hatred, derision, and bigotry in adults. From my experience, neither religiosity nor belief in a deity is a prerequisite for caring about other people. I lost friends when I left the church. I lost more when I declared my "atheism" because it meant I was no longer a "good person!" in many peoples' eyes.

Oh, come'on...That's so tolerant! I am still the same person. I am loyal and loving. We have raised kind and empathetic kids. I help other people with chronic illness. So, consequently, I do not believe in a special person in the sky who is a "god."

Humanist:

I believe all living humans are equal and should be treated with dignity, respect, equity, and should have equality. I think until that is a factual statement, we must make sure we are helping those who are facing current oppression or the after-effects of past oppression. Humanism includes being anti-racist, being against xenophobia, being a feminist, being an ally for the LGBTQIA+ community, and believing in complete religious freedom, including being pro-choice. Until we each have complete autonomy, including bodily autonomy, there is no freedom.

Spirituality:

Religion and spirituality are supposed to practice love, instead, we have people hating each other based upon their beliefs. I believe we have the -isms and -phobias, which often stem from white supremacy and separatist ideas rooted in religion. Hate stems from fear of change. These problems are part of what originally led me to leave religion and seek out spirituality, and now I have a very difficult time with any sort of spiritual teachings outside of my own study. You can be a super spiritual, loving, being, doing good in the world, and have it all be internally motivated instead of because of fear of a guy in the sky or hell or karma... or other punishment.

My spirituality is completely internal and comes from the ideas of equality and equity and love. It is based on the agape love of all humans, the earth, the universe, and nature as well as a personal understanding of my place in the universe rather than what someone tells me to believe.

Countless belief systems utilize some form of positive thinking, and it has been shown in studies about chronic illness to produce better outcomes. However, some in religion and spirituality have taken that too far. In TMT I spoke about my former boss (that was not at a church) who told me not to "speak" my illness aloud because that would "call it into existence" and that "I should claim healing by Jesus's stripes." She had no place to tell me I wasn't "doing" religion correctly as we didn't work in a religious environment. I wish I knew then that she was violating the law, but I didn't. Instead, I was young and allowed these words to make me feel ashamed and disconnected from "God." She made me feel I wasn't faithful enough otherwise God wouldn't have "forsaken" me and made me sick. What a bunch of bullshit.

Or take *The Secret*, it has been widely interpreted to put the onus of responsibility on the person for not thinking positively enough or meditating hard enough. This has gone mainstream and has caused so much guilt and shame in chronic illness circles. Just like we cannot pray it away, we cannot "meditate" or "deep breathe" autoimmune disease away. What we *can* do is use these things as *tools* for comfort and solace, and maybe grounding, which can all decrease stress and potentially help with symptoms. However, telling someone they didn't pray or think positively "hard enough" is a type of guilt and shame that is, in my opinion, manipulative, bordering on religious and spiritual abuse.

For instance, I once had someone tell me to stop saying, "I can't get off the floor," when they asked if I wanted to attend yoga class with them. Their reason was the statement was an energetically negative, "self-limiting belief." Now, I'm as much about positive self-talk as any other essential oil-using, incense burning, crystal wearing, earthy-tasting tea drinking, woo-woo 2020s hippie, and we use the power of positive thinking a lot throughout my family's life; but I was merely describing the literal truth of my physical condition: "I cannot get up from the floor."

Just like the aforementioned boss, this well-meaning person was telling me that acknowledging an authentic symptom of my disease, hip weakness and the inability to get up from the floor unassisted, would give it power over me. Yeah, sorry bro, that's not how it works!

When applied with love, religion and spirituality can bring comfort and hope, but neither change physical reality. Sometimes it comes down to a matter of physical ability, sometimes it is necessity, sometimes it is legitimate safety. My friend Keeya, who lives with mast cell activation syndrome, said, "With adrenal insufficiency if you don't respect 'can't,' you die."

Back when the yoga comment was made to me, Rickey and I had a good laugh about how I should positively reword, "I can't get off the floor.":

"My legs like the floor, I choose to stay here."

"The view is better down here; I think I'll stay awhile."

"I enjoy being lifted from the supine position."

"I'm stuck mother fucker!"

Or my personal favorite...short and sweet. "Fuck off!"

But honestly, the damage was done. I felt minimized, unheard, and dismissed. This person, someone who espoused inclusivity, love, and acceptance and who probably thought they were being encouraging, missed the mark. They completely ignored my physical limitation to push their spiritual agenda: "if you believe you can, you can do it." But...that is just not true and let's call it what it is. Ableist and harmful. Impact trumps intent!

Living as if we've entered *The Matrix,* "There is no spoon!"[12], may work in making dream boards and manifesting your most positive intentions, but it isn't going to make sickness go away. Even in manifesting your best life, the true teachings about positive thinking, as I understand them, are threefold.

#1 You set an intention.

#2 You align your thoughts and attitudes to that intention (as well as humanly possible, and when thoughts stray you bring them back to that intention).

#3 Finally, and equally as important, you take consistent action to work toward that reality.

A singer doesn't just say, "I am going to be a record-breaking music star," and then sit at home watching other singers on TV, forget about practicing, and wait for stardom to happen. They align their thoughts, intentions, and passion together with doing all *efforts* toward a music career for it to come to fruition.

THERE ARE VARYING LEVELS of "disability," as I mentioned before, mine is largely invisible. But I am not invisible, and neither is my communicated message when I share my limitations with others. People should be careful not to allow their religion or spirituality erase the person they are talking to. Yoga was, and still is, out of the question for me unless I modify it because, get this, I can't get up from the fucking floor alone! That is not a self-limiting belief. **It is Truth.**

How did we get to this point with the (new age) spirituality world which basically, among other things, grew out of a rejection of organized religion? This is just my opinion as a former participant and I want to be clear that I am talking about New Age Spirituality as a whole, not one person, and especially not Neale Donald Walsch who I believe to be clear-hearted and have never seen do any of the things discussed here.

I think people should be paid for their work, otherwise, how the heck are we, they, anyone supposed to pay their own bills? I am talking about people who cross the line into implanting fear and control. Unfortunately, I'm afraid as soon as any set of ideas starts to make money someone tries to codify it, make it indispensable to keep making money, keep amassing power, and followers. One of the ways to do that is to inject fear...in this case it was fear of not being positive enough.

In my opinion, these are some of the most dangerously applied ideas from *The Secret* and other self-help books. Using positivity as a tool is one thing, using it as a mechanism of fear and control, for instance, blaming someone for not being able to meditate themselves to be physically "well," is a completely different beast and antithetical to the original intent.

Aside from the fact that I felt ignored in the yoga situation and others, part of my loss of desire to participate in any spiritual practice outside my own family is the idea that someone outside of yourself can evaluate, calculate, or assess your words, your ideas, or your actions to see if you are "spiritual enough." Where does it end for fuck's sake? Spirituality teaches that you are "enough" as yourself, yet all these practices, in my experience, still fall into the trap of eventually, teaching you that you should fear not "being enough."

Spirituality's or religion's values in your life, or to be as clear as possible, your relationship with your deity or higher power, should be yours to assess alone. I've read about a lot of the world's religions in my search for the *meaning of life*. Most of the world's religions, including Christianity, were originally based on a personal relationship with the higher power. The human leaders are just supposed to be intermediaries and conduits. What's the problem with intermediaries? They are human. Eventually those humans own agendas and biases show up. Pride. Money. Power. Ego. Place of origin. Unconscious prejudice. Privilege. Then the ideals of the belief system start to get interpreted through their lenses.

We are all fallible but looking to another human to bring us our spirituality is where we set ourselves up to have others shame and guilt us for not meeting **their** expectations; expectations that often don't make sense because they aren't interpreting messages from a neutral place but from a place of an agenda. Everyone has an agenda. At all times.

Just as I do.

My agenda is trying to persuade you not to allow others to make you feel bad about yourself and your experiences of illness! It can be detrimental to anyone, and I personally believe it is why the world is in the state it is in. Collectively, we are no longer relying on our inner compass of how to treat each other according to a guiding principle of **love**. But this guilt and shame is particularly detrimental when it pertains to how that affects your place in, and view of, your illness and what it does in your life. It is antithetical to what is craved by people who are struggling with illness, and needing the balm of hope, peace, and support religion and spirituality could bring. This antithetical thing — call it guilt, shame, blame, whatever it is interpreted by the receiver as is making people who have illnesses feel alienated from their true selves. Many have told me privately in their hardest times of physical and emotional need that they feel neglected, ostracized, harmed and abandoned by their God or higher power because of the actions and words of humans.

It's sad that people seeking comfort and peace are not always getting it, and that is why I have walked away, twice, from the codified practice of spirituality.

Chapter 4
The Unrelenting Trauma of Being Sick

———

"Lovely," by Billie Eilish and Khalid

Trigger warning, talk about suicidal ideation in this chapter.

Having a cyclical, progressive, incurable, and untreatable chronic illness is inconvenient. It is traumatic. It is painful. It doesn't stop. It harms relationships. It can destroy your desired career and other plans. And that minimum is if you are lucky!

Some die early deaths. Some are left in emotional, physical, familial, and/or financial ruin. Some suffer in intractable pain with doctors who "don't believe" in the pain and are treated worse than we would knowingly treat anyone or any other living thing.

In the United States, we have people who are being denied health care, denied treatments, and denied dignity because of race, gender, gender identity, sexual orientation, or economic status. As high as 85% of people living unhoused[13] in the US have been found to have some type of chronic illness, including mental or physical. The high financial burden of being sick is not only traumatic, but also devastating. Some of the unhoused people could have gotten sick on the street, but they are then at higher risk and have less access for care. It is a vicious cycle of its own that is unAmerican. Why are any of us, housed or unhoused seen as lesser than? Why do we deserve less consideration? And why does illness mean we have all other parts of our lives at risk for devastation?

Even people who are financially secure and have private insurance from their family member's job or their own job suffer from inadequate care. Insurance often does whatever it can to deny, delay, and second-guess care. The problem with this is that patients should be thinking about our health, taking care of ourselves, resting, eating healthful foods, resting, managing our doctor's appointments, resting, and enjoying our families when we have the energy. Instead, we spend countless hours on the phone with insurance companies fighting with them, appealing ridiculous decisions, being go-betweens with them and medical providers; all because the insurance companies have decided that they know more than the specialists. I just read a disturbing account of a young man with ulcerative colitis whose insurance company appears to have deliberately ignored medical advice, from The Mayo Clinic (experts in his disease) and their own hired experts.[14] The only reason their callousness was exposed was because his family sued them, and the records were subpoenaed. Their employees are on recorded lines laughing, making fun of his family, lying about expert conversations, and hiding documents to save money. SICK! I might even say this behavior is sicker than I am.

Now, keep in mind that dermatomyositis has three main areas of specialty, and other areas that are called in for ancillary problems caused by DM.

The main areas are dermatology, rheumatology, and neurology (specifically neuro-muscular neurologists). There are a number of life-saving medications which have been shown to work for DM in peer-reviewed studies and are widely used in practice but are considered off-label use because of the arduous process to be "FDA-approved." I have had various insurance companies throughout the years tell me that my claims for them have been denied by nurses, OBGYNs, dentists, and pharmacists, none of whom specialize in my disease. Let me make something clear...there are neurologists, dermatologists, and rheumatologists who have never treated dermatomyositis and cannot even pronounce it. It is highly suspect that any one of those specialties at the insurance company producing denials know more than my own doctors.

Most recently, it is highly suspect and is offensive, that the people at the insurance company pretend to know more than my dermatologist who studied under one of the foremost experts in dermatomyositis...The gall to insert themselves between patient and doctor knows no bounds. It is funny that once I mentioned that to the appeals department on a recorded line, and pointed out that the medication is mentioned in dozens (over 100) of peer reviewed studies to reduce DM skin presentation, and nerve and skin pain within days, my denied prescription was reconsidered and approved within 30 minutes (not nearly enough time for them to have contacted that doctor to make any clarifications — and he verified later that they did not).

A few weeks later another one told me "footcare" is only covered for patients with diabetes. I have Raynaud's and neuropathy. At the time, I had horrible infections in my (multiple) in-grown toenails and they denied the initial visit to a foot doctor/podiatrist because I'm not diabetic and, according to them, only diabetics have medical necessity for footcare unless you get a prior authorization.

I had checked to see if the doctor was in-network on the website, there was no asterisk to say, "check policy for medical necessity." There was not footnote (no pun intended) to say that the doctor was only covered for diabetes. Let's be clear, there are many other conditions that affect foot health, to the potential detriment of your health and the risk of your life aside from diabetes. I asked how to get a PA for medical necessity for footcare without seeing a foot doctor...they couldn't answer...and in fact after I asked multiple times for clarifications rather than for her to read the statement over and over, the representative started to shout at me. I told her to stop yelling and transfer me. The next person gave me the proper info to give my doctor to correct the claim to show medical necessity and my claim was paid.

As I mentioned earlier in the conversation with Sage, I think I should start to keep track of my time on the phone with the insurance company explaining their job to them and send them a monthly bill. I wonder if that would change the ways in which they operate.

Insurance should be there to do the job of paying for medical care as outlined by the doctor and agreed upon by the patient. It should not be the cause of more stress, and it certainly should not be the arbiter of who gets to live and die, which insurance companies sometimes seem to take on as a part of their rights; especially when supplanting themselves between patient and doctor.

SOME OF US BEGIN LIVING in this cyclic and never-ending limbo of better-worse-improvement-decline-oddity-novelty-help-neglect-belief-disbelief that we never asked for and wouldn't wish on anyone. I recently read about a newer classification of Post-Traumatic Stress Disorder, with the word "complex" added to the beginning of it (C-PTSD) in which it looks at the damage of long-term, sustained abuse or traumatic situations. I had previously heard of people getting diagnosed with a type of PTSD based on chronic health conditions. Admittedly, I am not a doctor or psychiatrist, but I am a professional **patient**. By now I think I could convincingly play a doctor on Grey's Anatomy. Although one source I read about C-PTSD[15] specifically says it relates to ongoing "relational trauma" (meaning from another person) I can't say for sure, but when I read about C-PTSD, I can't help but think the trauma of the never-ending cycle of pain and suffering autoimmune and other chronic illness patients experience sounds like ongoing and sustained trauma. That trauma has to alter our brains and body chemistry. I know mine has been. For an in-depth discussion about chronic illness-induced PTSD please read this sourced article on *The Mighty*.[16] However, I want to make it very clear that this is not a reason to minimize, demean, or otherwise belittle any patient's physical illness. More on that in Chapter 11.

In 2021, I was trying a new medication, a Jak inhibitor. I took exactly four pills, one per day, for four days. On the second day we noticed I had become weepy, saying things like, "I wish I wasn't such a burden." But Scott and I weren't alarmed, *being sick sucks*, and I have mentioned feeling like a burden to him before. However, it has always been undergirded with gratitude for his care and love. He grabbed my hand and said his usual, "you aren't a burden, I love you, we are good," refrain; and we moved on. On the third day, and in hindsight, we should have taken notice of this, I asked him "Would you be better off without me?" He said, "Of course not, why would you ask that?"

I said something like, "I must just be exhausted and tired of these meds and worried this one won't work." Since I had no other warning signs or major mental illness history to be concerned about, we didn't really think any more of it and went about the day.

After four pills, it was a Monday, November 1, 2021. I was driving home from dropping my daughter off and saw a guardrail with a cliff. I heard something in my head, it felt distant, but it was *definitely* inside me, say or feel, (that part is very hard to explain), "You could drive off that cliff or into that guardrail right now. It would be over in a split second, and they wouldn't have to take care of you anymore, life would be so much easier for everyone else."

I'm telling you; the entire thought was less than a millisecond long.

Thankfully, another part of my brain immediately kicked in. Maybe it was a part of my brain that knew about pharmacology from working at a children's home part-time with mentally ill children in my 20s or from working as a psych tech in the psychiatric ward right after college. Maybe it was the part of me that worked with women in recovery in a court-mandated drug treatment program or had interned in the women's prison in college working with a similar population of women.

Either way some part of me knew that there was some chemical misfiring in my brain. It probably worked along with the part of my brain that works so hard to stay alive. Whatever part or parts of my brain kicked in, in that millisecond, it or they said, "what the fuck?" and automatically pressed dial on my phone and called Scott before I even passed the guardrail.

I sobbed into the phone, telling him what happened, and asked him to talk to me until I got some coffee — *at a coffee shop* (thinking the chemicals must be messed up in my brain and coffee would change them) — because I didn't even trust myself to go home alone at the time. I was afraid if I went home, I wouldn't make coffee and without something to quickly change my brain chemicals I wouldn't be safe. After I had the coffee, I called Jaime, my best friend who, thankfully, stayed on FaceTime with me for **four hours** until I felt safe. Scott would have come home if it weren't for her, obviously, but thankfully, she was able to be with me, virtually, until every last bit of that scary feeling passed. My doctor and I agreed to stop the medicine, and I made a report to the drug company and the FDA.

There are only a handful of prior reports (I think there were a maximum of 10 official reports at that point) of this happening on that particular drug (and some additional reports of adolescents with suicidal ideation and attempts in an actual study) but it made me wonder, how many times do we hear of someone ending their lives, seemingly out of the blue? I worry about how close I was to becoming one of those statistics and how many people have this happen and complete the suicide because they do not understand that the thought is happening due to the medication changing their brain? It is scary sitting here remembering it, but it was worse than anything I've ever experienced that day.

This is a good place to remind you of the suicide hotline: 988lifeline.org or dial 988 in the US. Had Scott and Jaime not been available that day I would have called 911 or called the suicide hotline as 988 wasn't around yet.

DURING A SUBSEQUENT, long-term, ongoing, uncontrolled skin flare, my managing doctor called me back at the **best** time imaginable, while I was picking up my medication in Target. I do not have the best phone reception in my town, so I had no choice but to stay still for 45 minutes to talk to him in the middle of the children's clothing section (the most private place I could find without dropping his call) to discuss my recent colonoscopy and endoscopy in which the GI doctor found evidence of my Dermatomyositis rash inside my gut.

There I was, bawling, sobbing, and snotting into my KN-95 mask (I am an "ugly crier," so it was gross!), as I begged him to figure out how to help me because I felt like I was losing me, was going to lose Scott, and really, was losing "IT!". In that year since I had moved to Minnesota, we have re-tried multiple meds from the past 20+ years and stopped them, again, due to them failing to help or due to side effects (mood swings, migraines, rashes, or shingles). I told him I am not myself. I am short, scratch that, I am mean at times, with my husband and daughter due to the frustration and pain. The steroid pulses we were trying on infusion nights were not metabolizing out as expected. I was again enduring "roid rage" and some loss of reality. They have made me curt (not me) and led to me making some terrible statements to Scott (who, if you have read TMT or followed my posts/previous blogs, you know is an absolute angel, my soulmate and love of all my infinite lives) and being extremely snappy with Sage, my sweet girl who has been through so much as a child of a sick mom.

So back to my doctor and I having our heart-to-heart in Target...we were discussing all of this, and he said what I believe is the single most important thing any doctor has ever said to me. It made me feel less "not okay" and out of control than I had been feeling for weeks.

I'm paraphrasing, but he basically said, *"Emily, you are not losing it. Anyone...anyone who has been at this as long as you have with refractory skin lesions, cyclical muscle weakness, fatigue, pain, and everything else plus so many failed medications and side effects, would be feeling helpless, alone, and hopeless. But I am here. Scott is here. And neither of us is going anywhere. Scott knows you didn't mean anything you said under those stupid steroids. He knows you better than that. Let's get this new medication approved and see if we can get you relief."*

I've had some shitty doctors and I've had some amazing doctors. Two doctors that I cried to leave when we moved away from Missouri. But I have never felt so seen, understood, and so protected as I did in that moment, which of course made the tears fall all the more.

PS. The new medication to which he referred was another Jak-inhibitor. Yep, I tried another one a year after the first and apparently, I am unable to take them at all. Three weeks in, I also developed suicidal thoughts. This was after we did an eight-day pseudo-suicide-watch while I got used to the medicine. Scott worked from home the week of Thanksgiving (2022) and I did okay, except that I was having a terrible time waking up, I was hungrier than I could ever imagine, and I broke out in a rash on the 10th day. We took a couple of days to back off and retry and it seemed okay until the third week when it suddenly hit me in a conversation with Scott that I didn't want to live anymore. I stopped myself from voicing it initially, then I got scared and confessed that I had another *initial* suicidal thought, but not actively wanting to hurt myself, more along the lines of questioning why I was still alive and how much of a burden I was, as well as how much easier it would be if I was "gone"...the first sign we had missed from a year before. I asked him to work from home the next day so I wouldn't be alone until we spoke to my doctor, and I skipped my next dose. (These actions were pre-planned in case I had a recurrence of the suicidal thoughts.) We stopped the medication, and my chart now says I cannot take Jak-inhibitors going forward. Reports were made again to the drug company and FDA.

I'm grateful we had those preliminary conversations and knew how to handle if it came up again.

JUST TO PROVE THAT the trauma of this fucking disease is unrelenting, I saw another specialist for one of my other conditions a couple months later. I had to go through the whole suicidal ideation — side effect story again. I made it clear that my main DM doctor, my husband, and I had things under control and that I am **not** suicidal. But ... he freaked out anyway and claimed I couldn't have had SI without having it lurking undetected ready to come out. What a crock of shit, it was a side effect. He told me he *had to refer me back to my PCP to ask for a psych eval.* Keep in mind, this is three months after the incident. This is after my DM specialist and I had worked through all the scenarios. This is after we had assured ourselves for months(!) that I am safe. But since I mentioned that I am tired of the unrelentingness of the meds not working and he flipped. I got a call the next day from my PCP for a meeting. I delayed it by a week so I could talk with my DM specialist first with Scott in attendance. We reviewed our information and my status. I went to the PCP meeting with my plan in place, I refused the psych eval and gave my reasons, including that I am well-adjusted, well-taken care of, have access to therapy **when I need it**, and am unable to take psych meds anyway due to a history of side effects detrimental to my heart from when I took various ones for my raynauds. Plus, I reminded my PCP that this was a gross overreaction that minimizes the root problem, we are not finding appropriate medication to treat my DM and my DM doctor and I are working on this. My PCP agreed to drop it.

Now, I do not have a problem with psychiatric care as a whole. I think it is important when warranted, but do not send me there because you do not understand side effects and the effects that medications have on the brain. Do not further traumatize me when I just came through one of the scariest things that could happen, my brain being told by a medication to kill me and survived it because of preparation and vigilance. Do not minimize our vigilance and my word when I tell you I am safe; when I am telling you I need help with my physical health, the part you are an expert in. That is the worst thing you can do to a person struggling to manage chronic illness.

Another untenable part of this experience is I have learned that the people who make my disease about themselves don't belong in my life. I have had a couple of relatives who would get angry if they called me and I didn't return their call immediately when I didn't feel up to talking. They thought it meant I was in the hospital too sick to talk. Dude, I'm pretty sure if I'm that acutely ill, someone will let you know. In order to preserve the relationships, I avoided talking about my health altogether and tried to enjoy our time in other ways. That didn't work! I was told I was being secretive and hiding that I was about to die...as if I needed to hear that!

Their questions got more persistent, to the point of intrusive. Then they started to lay guilt trips on me about how much their worry about my illness affected them. Unfortunately, this is a recurring theme in my life, other people's negative emotional stress about me and my disease being pushed onto me, however all this conversation does is cause **me** stress and compounded guilt because it isn't like I can change my circumstance. I cannot wish myself better to assuage someone else's fears. Quite frankly it isn't my responsibility to do so anyway. I understand this is coming from a somewhat misguided place of love and caring, but they need to process their grief and fears about my health status with someone else, not me, the sick person. My disease is not about you.

Note: I have heard that this has happened over and over to other people with chronic illness as well, so it isn't isolated to my family.

The bottom line is that we have to learn to advocate for ourselves in all avenues of our lives, even the toughest ones, even from the doctors because while they may be the medical expert, you are the expert on your own body. That means confronting the hard truths of what the autoimmune abyss does to you, your relationships, and your life. You have to be able to be honest with those around you and if something isn't working be willing to say, "nope" and move on. It's hard but worth it. There are support networks out there. As I've mentioned before I've been in and out of therapy throughout my adulthood because sometimes the overwhelm is too much. There are support groups for many of the diseases. Often your friends want to be there for you, you just have to ask for exactly what it is that you need.

Chapter 5

At Least You Don't Have...

[Insert Disease Someone Thinks Is Worse Here]!

———

"Superman (It's not easy)," by Five for Fighting

Let's get this out of the way. Dermatomyositis and many other autoimmune diseases can be fatal [some immediate, some down the road]. Most doctors will casually tell an autoimmune patient, "At least you don't have cancer," (more on this one later), "you won't die from myositis/autoimmune disease, but maybe from a complication from it" or "you won't die from myositis, but you will die with it."

Okay, I'm sorry, what the hell do any of those things mean?

In 2003, when I was finally diagnosed, 7-8 years after I developed the acute symptoms, the prognosis was confusing. There were varying timelines quoted and in my research between "not fatal" and 5-15 years.

If I had already beaten the first layer of that prognosis (I'd survived the "already dead" to "five years" phases) did that mean I wouldn't die? If I hadn't yet developed cancer, heart disease, perforated bowels, lung involvement, did that mean I wouldn't? Does having (suspected) Juvenile onset-dermatomyositis change that picture? (Quick note, juvenile-onset can be terrible and/or fatal too. I do not want to minimize its horrible impact, even if treated correctly, sometimes it is refractory and children suffer greatly.)

If I had never heard of the disease and most medical professionals hadn't either, how was I ever going to get adequate care? Who knows?! The doctors sure do not!

...and come on...let's be real...do we really want to have our barometer for the value and quality of someone's life with chronic illness be "not cancer" when they are taking cancer drugs anyway and dealing with chemo side effects? Do we want the bar to be "not bedridden?" Should the measure of success be "not dead?"

What a load of horse shit. I refuse to accept any of them as the best I can get.

I am not diminishing anyone's cancer journey, or any other horrible disease for that matter, and I fear getting that diagnosis *added* to my own as much as anyone else thinks about the "big C" — but let's do and be better, shall we? My quality of life, and the rest of the people in the chronic illness and autoimmune community, all deserve to be better than waiting to die from a blood clot, or a misfiring of a chemical in my brain due to a medication side effect that makes me drive off a cliff after four pills, or pneumonia, or ILD (interstitial lung disease), or heart failure, or myositis-related cancer...etc.

I recently read an Instagram post explaining how we feel when having a chronic illness. The writer talked about the feeling that once you don't get better people seem to get impatient or just move on.[17] This is something I think I've heard from many of my chronic illness friends, is that although many types of chronic illness are devastating, rare diseases are not taken as seriously as ones that are more well known, and as such we are expected to be okay within some magical amount of time.

However, I am a firm believer in the idea that whatever health crisis is happening to YOU is the most important thing happening to YOU at that moment. I don't believe in measuring pain. I don't think it is useful to get out a suffering stick and say, "Emily's had myositis her whole adult life" and therefore my loved ones should keep their suffering to themselves. I have had countless people express guilt to me after complaining about life's problems whether it be family issues, work-related, or illness.

First, I take anyone confiding in me as a moment of trust and respect. It is an honor to be taken into confidence. Second, when they express that guilt, "oh I shouldn't complain to you, you are so sick and don't feel well." I am not perfect, but I always try to answer something like, "whatever is happening to you is just as big and important to you in this moment, as anything that happens to anyone else, please do not diminish it because of me. I want to be here for you."

Unfortunately, society doesn't always give chronic illness sufferers the same respect.

Chapter 6

Medical Personnel Can't Pronounce Dermatomyositis

But Think They Know Me

I've got news for you Mr. Doctor What's Your name, You Don't Know Me!

If you have ever had, or read about, an out-of-body experience, you may be familiar with how it feels to walk into an ER for help with something like a high heart rate or blood pressure, a new symptom, pain, anything that has to do with your rare disease, or something that isn't easy to solve and be told to see a psychiatrist, that you are a drug seeker, or a faker. This isn't an accident. The medical community has been conditioned to disbelieve and dismiss patients in pain, chronic illness sufferers, and people with complex cases. Sorry, peeps, especially women with chronic illness.

I would further challenge this understanding of the medical community and suggest that some of it, for some of the practitioners who are particularly vicious, amounts to intentional dismissal. That dismissal could result from being jaded or from being overworked, but honestly, that's not my, or any other patient's, problem! We don't want to be there, being difficult to figure out, any more than you want us to be!

Ask chronic illness patients who face doctors on a routine basis, especially when we encounter physicians in odd circumstances such as emergency rooms. I don't think this is merely a matter of lack of knowledge. I think some of it, unfortunately, moves into willful ignorance. As I am finishing the finals edits, I came across a piece on *The Mighty* in which a fellow chronic illness patient describes a similar experience.[19] At some point the Medical community must listen.

Most disturbingly, in the US, if one is typically in a "class" widely understood to be "vulnerable" then walking into any doctor's office can be scary because you do not know what extremism you may be facing. I speak from my own experience as a woman with chronic illness, but also from listening and hearing the horrendous treatment of others with chronic illness who have been ignored, dismissed, and mistreated. I am willing to be corrected as I am not speaking solely from my own experience, but I have heard from, and of, people who are mistreated because they are, in no particular order: Black women, women of color, poor women and poor men, trans women, trans Black women, trans women of color, white women, trans men, non-binary people, openly gay and bi men, openly gay and bi women, people who speak a language other than English, non-Christian people, and so many other people who may qualify as "different" or "new" "or "non-conforming" to the medical person standing before them.

This isn't a new topic, but I would be remiss to fail to mention that Black people were still being *unethically* experimented on by so-called reputable medical institutions up until the 1990s.[20] The Tuskegee medical experiments only ended in 1972, by the US government! That is really not that long ago....and these are the studies we **know** about.

Black women who are sick are still disbelieved at much higher rates than any other segment of the population. Dermatological disease photos are still mostly catalogued with light-colored skin. A Black medical student named Malone Mukwende started a project in 2020 to ensure Black skin is included in dermatology photos[21] because if doctors do not know what a rash looks like on darker skin how can it be diagnosed? Black bodies are still underrepresented in medical literature and textbooks.[22]

It is disgusting to know it has taken this long to put attention on BIPOC medical abuse. Our entire society is complicit. The systemic problems can only continue when non-marginalized people no longer stay silent alongside all our chronic illness siblings. I encourage all of us with chronic illness, and the care partners who support us, to learn about the abuses of all people with chronic illness and speak up to stand in unity with all who need equitable, fair, and acceptable care. None of us are okay when all of us are not okay.

BACK TO THE ER

I can't tell you how many times I have gone into an ER for pain or a scary new symptom, with a list of drug allergies that includes the majority of opioids and been counseled on drug seeking by a doctor who needed me to explain what dermatomyositis is, much less how to pronounce it.

Excuse me. What drug do you believe I seek, jerk? I can't take most of them. I want you to figure out *why* I am in pain or *why* I have something wrong no one in the normal world has ever heard of, give me some immediate relief — usually a bag of fluids, a shot of Toradol (which is a strong anti-inflammatory), bring my heart rate and BP down — and make sure nothing is immediately life-threatening.

The thing is, it takes a lot for someone like me — immune suppressed and living in immense pain every single day of my life — to go into the germ-infested petri dish that the rest of the world calls the ER. I didn't come in lightly. My braving the So-Called Emergency room means I'm in a, well, EMERGENCY, and I'd like a little relief or reassurance rather than your judgment. Plus, I have so many weird things going on with my and inside my body at all times that it takes a lot for me to think I should even go in. While the conventional wisdom is "new or worsening shooting chest pain" means get checked out, I would be at the ER every other week for worsening, unidentified chest pain. I get it, they don't know why. What if sometime I ignore it and it's the wrong time?

Many times, the ER attendings come in with a gaggle of medical students and residents who think it's "so cool" or "wow, rad" to see my open, exposed, plaque-filled rash. "Fuck all the way off" ... seriously. It was "cool" for about the first 30 medical students.

Here is a teaching moment for attendings: 1) ask my permission before bringing in the residents and medical students, even if it is just as a courtesy and you intend to bring them anyway. 2) take a moment and teach the residents and medical students to talk about how "cool" my rash looks after they leave the room (didn't they watch any hospital TV shows before becoming a doctor?)! I don't need to hear it. I'd like a little bit of decorum from my "doctors," kind of like how I like a little bit of salt on my French fries!

Back to know-it-all-doctors who know nothing about my conditions, a couple of years ago, during the height of the Covid pandemic, an ER doctor, if I recall correctly his name was Dr. Asshat, told me that my, later to be diagnosed, autonomic dysfunction/dysautonomia/orthostatic hypotension/POTS, was a major undiagnosed psychiatric illness. It was like before I was diagnosed with dermatomyositis all over again. He told me my heart symptoms were psychosomatic. They were not. The elevated heart rate and erratic blood pressure were real.

Earlier, I had been sitting, socially distanced, on the porch with my neighbor and suddenly had severe chest pain and shortness of breath, with an elevated pulse and blood pressure. I kept clutching my chest, thinking I was just hot and having an asthma attack from the heat. She told me I was turning grey and after having me text Scott to come outside, she called 911. The paramedics decided I should go to the hospital, due to my health and family history. The first ER doc I saw ordered tests before going off shift and was adamant we did the right thing coming in; he would rather see someone 1000 times with these symptoms and (hopefully) have them come back with clear tests than ignore it once with a tragic result.

The second doctor, Dr. Asshat, is the one who came in with my clear test results and proceeded to tell me I should be on multiple psychiatric meds. He basically said I was faking for attention. I looked at Scott and in the calmest voice I could muster, realizing this dude could commit me for a multi-day psych eval since he had already made up his mind, asked as calmly and nicely as possible (not easy for me at the time), "Are you aware of dermatomyositis and the heart implications that indicate advanced stage disease?" He replied, "Uh, well, kind of, I mean, yes, but that's not the problem here. You are exhibiting signs of stress and psychiatric illness that would take multiple medications to control."

Me, in my calmest, nicest, I-refuse-to-go-off-on-this-contemptable-assface-and-give-him-what-he-wants-voice, possible: "Cool, thanks, I'm pretty sure my GP and I are more aware of my condition than you, since you didn't even pronounce D-E-R-M-A-T-O-M-Y-O-S-I-T-I-S correctly, and I am getting scheduled for dysautonomia testing, but just release me and I'll talk to her." He tried to *flex* and argue his point but I gritted my teeth, for once, and said "thanks for your help, please release me" ...and got the **fuck outta there.**

A couple of quick notes:

#1 Mental illness is nothing for which to be ashamed. It is as medical as IBS. We need to destigmatize it. Period. More about this in Chapter 11.

#2. For various reasons, I've been in therapy many of the years since I was 18. I think all adults should avail themselves of therapy whether they have chronic illness, trauma, relationship issues in their past, present, or none of the above. It is a great conduit of self-discovery.

#3 Mental illness of the type of which he was attempting to "diagnose" me, especially within the context of over two and a half decades of chronic illness attacking my body, is not something he was qualified to call in the ER. Situational anxiety is not uncommon in chronic illness, but that is not what he was referring to and it was not what was happening.

#4 We texted my therapist's emergency number on our way home and thankfully she was available to talk...we told her about Dr. Asshat. She agreed what he had done was inexcusable and incorrect. She gave me reassurance that I couldn't manufacture the symptoms that we all knew I had been noticing for weeks and that some doctors just get it wrong.

#5 When I spoke to my GP the next day, she was appalled at the treatment I received, I'll leave it at that.

Less than a week later I was woken up in the middle of the night by an elevated BP and tachycardia. Scott and I did all the techniques we knew to attempt to get it down with no success. We called 911 who also couldn't determine why my heart was going haywire. Thankfully Dr. Asshat wasn't on duty.

At first, that night's doc kept telling me that after giving me meds to help me rest (and fall asleep) that my heart rate only went up when they walked into the room and woke me up – OMG, you can't make this ignorant shit up — of course it goes up when you startle someone awake! After I pointed this out and the fact that I was awaiting confirmation of testing for dysautonomia (autonomic dysfunction) they tested and released me with metoprolol, which miraculously had brought my heart rate and BP to normal, along with the fluids and sleep.

Autonomic dysfunction was definitively diagnosed a couple weeks later by a tilt table test. I still take the metoprolol, now, over three years later to control the tachycardia. I also take Pedialyte every morning and additional times on bad days. When I have tried to decrease the heart medicine or Pedialyte, the tachycardia and blood pressure issues come back with a vengeance. For those who don't know, one of the main ways to treat dysautonomia, especially the parts of it involving the heart are to increase fluids and add electrolytes. As I'm writing this it occurs to me, probably for the first time, that the reason I got immediate relief from the tachycardia and fluctuating BP upon getting an IV is the fluids! Why isn't that on the doctors' radar? POTS is a type of dysautonomia, it's not that rare.

Ugh. The frustration continues and I hear of so many other people who face similar situations of dismissal and denial by the very doctors who should be caring for them, rather than treating us as if we are there by choice; because yes, my choice is to spend the day in an ER with germs swirling around me when I could be at home with my family...especially compounded by nurses and doctors telling me I am a hypochondriac. Give me a fucking break.

BETTER ACCEPTANCE OF treatment for mental illness and increased understanding of mental health is very important. If I actually had a mental illness that would be helped with ongoing medication, and didn't cause additional harm, I would agree immediately. But dismissing my very real physical symptoms because a doctor, especially Dr. Asshat, saw my voluminous chart and saw that my GP and I had discussed an anti-depressant was belittling and disrespectful. Besides, if he looked further into my drug profile, as he should have done, he would have also seen that I am adamantly averse to taking more medications than needed due to a history of terrible side effects and adverse reactions. Doctors minimizing symptoms of documented physical illness as a psychiatric break does nothing to destigmatize mental illness. This is abusive and detrimental to all patients. Full stop.

For instance, and when it applies to the above-mentioned, possibly well-meaning, but wildly misinformed, jerk: While I was there for a rapid heartbeat, anti-depressants (tricyclics, SSRIs, and SARIs) also make me tachycardic and hallucinate. Anti-anxiety meds or sedatives and sleeping pills, as well as anti-convulsant and nerve pain medications also make me hallucinate and have weird, violent dreams in which I am "locked-in." I also had this happen with Low-Dose Naltrexone (LDN) a drug that is typically used for withdrawal from opioids at high doses, but in low doses can help with pain and sleep, as well as, some people believe, inflammation, in people with chronic inflammatory diseases. LDN helped me for a very long time, except for the "locked-in" dreams.

"Locked-in" dreams, in my case — always nightmares — mean I know that I know I am dreaming but cannot get out. At some point, another part of my brain starts to try to bypass the locked-in dreams and in them, I start to create trap doors, open windows, and magic doors. The weird thing is sometimes those doors work and sometimes they don't. Eventually even if the medication is helping its intended use, the tachycardia, locked-in dreams, or other effects make it impossible to continue the drug.

I recently spoke to a long-time friend who also lives with multiple autoimmune diseases. She also, like me, tells it straight up like it is, often with colorful language. There is a reason I love her so much! I told her I was writing this follow-up book and that one of the chapters would entail all the shitty things doctors say to minimize or ignore our true experiences. She gave me permission to share this story.

Recently she was diagnosed with an additional autoimmune disease, I think this is her third one; it isn't unusual for these conditions to multiply like little fucking gremlins when given water. Earlier in her disease journey a doctor, I guess, actually understanding that intractable pain is often a feature of autoimmune disease, suggested that anti-depressants may help with her horrible pain. This is not an abnormal tactic, and is something I, and many other patients have tried with varying success and failure. Doctors will often claim that it will also do double-duty, helping with the emotional strain of chronic illness. It didn't help with the pain, but it gave her a sense of manufactured euphoria...Viv says to me, "I walked in for my next appointment and the doctor asks, 'So how are you feeling, is the antidepressant helping?'" In true Viv fashion she says, "'I guess so, because now I'm just sooo happy I feel like fucking shit!' He cracked up. Then I told him that I couldn't even cry anymore, and I used to cry while watching Lassie. I've been on antidepressants off and on for the past 20 years. If I wasn't on one and saw a new doctor, it's the very first thing they would want to prescribe, even though I told them I didn't think they helped. It's the first thing they want to do when they see a middle or older aged female come in with multiple complaints!" And no, it didn't really help her pain...but he didn't seem to think changes were needed to move forward. Again, another patient felt dismissed!

Since I'm complaining about ER docs, I should relay my most recent ER experience. I went in for dehydration because my body has, unfortunately, started rejecting my beloved SCIG. We have a love-hate relationship. I love the results but hate the side effects. SCIG loves to torture me. Anyway, I'll spare you the shitty blahs, but after weeks of barely being able to eat anything but soup, becoming overly familiar with my bathroom, and losing a few too many pounds for sustained health; I was dehydrated enough to get a fever and chills for the second time in two weeks. We headed to the ER and met a lovely doctor about our age who took me seriously. He ordered a load of tests and ran an IV of fluids to replenish me.

He came in later in the evening and asked if we minded talking to him about my experiences with dermatomyositis. He had a little familiarity with it and wanted to express his empathy for what I was going through as he knew enough to know it was a hard disease to have. We were very impressed as he asked me about my symptoms, diagnosis timeline, difficulties, and prior medications. He was very appreciative of our time because he said it would help him when he encounters patients with dermatomyositis in the future; we in turn expressed our own appreciation, both for his empathy and listening when we got there — he really paid attention and was responsive — and also that he cared enough, once I was feeling better and almost ready to leave to inquire more from me to help other patients in the future. This is what good doctors do.

Regardless of a medical person's intentions, treating chronic illness sufferers with such dismissal like from the earlier doctors, whether it is with prejudice and bias and/or as drug seekers or as fakers, or acting like there is a magic pill that will solve all their problems but not address the real issue, they do a great disservice to us. Really and truly, if we want to be honest, why does the medical community think it is okay to treat anyone with disgust? Many are clearly overworked, but medically compromised people are overwrought, whether they are chronically ill, mentally ill, addicted to drugs, or any other ailment and we **all** deserve to be treated with dignity, respect, and expediency. It doesn't take much to treat a person as a human being.

Unfortunately, the medical community is sometimes lacking in compassion and empathy, especially when speaking of the gatekeepers. Moreover, ironically, the compassion and empathy can really seem to lack when it comes to the hard cases, the ones of us who need it the most.

Chapter 7
What "I Just Can't Take It Anymore" Really Means

———

"Her Diamonds," by Rob Thomas

The thing with having a multi system disease that is unknown, rare, cyclical, intractable, refractory, and has no or few effective accepted treatments is everything is always a pain in the ass. It being an "invisible" rare disease also means that unless you come close to see my rash (oh, how people feel the right to comment on that rash! More on that later...), or know me well, you may think I seem like a "normal" or "healthy" person. There have been times that I needed a rollator/walker or cane, but fortunately I do not need assistive devices right now.

Please do not be mistaken, that doesn't mean I am in remission. I'm not cured. I am not fixed. I am not "okay." I exist. I live. I function on a basic level due to meds, the loving care of my husband, and the encouragement of my kids and other loved ones. Even with their love and support, I do not know how much more I can take; I'm exhausted and I do not know how much more I can take of this. I don't know how much more (fight? upmf? gumption? will? energy?) I have left. Sage asked me to stop saying this around her, because even though it is not suicidal and I am not giving up, it sounds that way to her. So, I try not to say it near her, but it is my truth; and it is a truth I hear over and over from others with all kinds of incurable, yet chronic diseases. What the hell are we supposed to do? How the fuck are we supposed to feel? There is nothing we can do. No where we can go. No promising end to the pain and tiredness and sometimes we feel defeated. Sometimes we need to allow ourselves to express the utterly complete devastation and futility we feel when we stare into this hopeless abyss every fucking day.

I mean, I am okay, some days, but some days I am far from okay. Some days I am "okay" half the day and writhing on the couch or in bed in pain the other half. Some days I can take care of myself in the morning and by the time Scott gets home from work I need him to undress me. Some days I have trouble waking up, literally, he shakes me until my brain will jolt awake, and then in the evening I sing and entertain them at dinner. Some days I am a shell of who I am and who I want to be, who I believe myself to be, and I sit, staring at the TV all day, in my pajamas, hair and teeth unbrushed, counting the hours until I will no longer be alone because the shaking, weakness, pain, and mental fog are so bad I do not want to walk more than a few feet at a time, afraid of falling or dropping something. Some days I wake up feeling *alive*, help Sage get ready for her day and as soon as she walks out the door, collapse into a heap of nothingness, only to be awoken by Scott's daily text, "coming home," completely unaware that the hours have passed. Some days, I can go watch Sage skate, grab lunch, or even go to a store alone (usually not all of those in one day, alone).

The day after my shots and infusions are the worst. I'm clumsier. I'm foggier. When we are making and packing Sage's breakfast and lunch before she leaves for the day I have more accidents in the kitchen. I drop things more easily. I can't cut her kiwi because I cut myself...on kiwi! What? Kiwi, one of the softest things to cut. I trip over my own feet more when walking through the kitchen. I spill more. While I pre-cook her lunch (or later dinner) the spatula flips out of my hand splattering me with grease and spraying food all over the floor, me, my clothes, and the stove and countertop. I forget what I am doing in the middle of a task.

Moreover, at times, I become useless. Smells of her food, food we make every day make me gag. I have to leave the kitchen until certain things are packed, or trash has to be taken out that is fresh and would normally not bother me. I spill hot water on me or her and burn one of us. I trip over the dog. I repeat myself...repeatedly. I cry because I feel inept and helpless. I am a highly educated, intelligent human and I can't remember how to pour milk.

Furthermore, I am subjecting my beautiful daughter to this. She is now almost eighteen, and while she has lived it her whole life, she is internalizing it differently. From a more adult perspective, but still my little girl, still my baby, but now in a grown-up body with a more grown-up mind, she has to see me and feel the pain differently because I can't hide it with a joke anymore. Sometimes she gets angry, sometimes she cries hard. How can I keep making her see me like this? What other choice is there? There isn't one.

We just keep going.

I fall.

I cry.

Someone picks me up.

I cry.

I keep going.

Chapter 8

No Dear, I'm Not Faking Being Sick, I'm Faking Being Well

"Fight Song," by Rachel Platten

I'm going to attempt to list some of the most ridiculous, unbelievable, hard-to-explain symptoms that I encounter as I move through life. These are the things that are what make up the unbearable abyss I stare into and why it gets overwhelming even if from the outside I "seem" to be doing okay; sometimes even to those closest to me. I hesitated to include this chapter. I almost deleted it after I wrote it, because I kept thinking, "people will think I'm a whiner." And "Why will anyone care about the details of the shit symptoms I endure?"

Then I remembered my promise to Connie. I would share it all. Not for sympathy, but because too many people are afraid to talk about it *aloud* — people are afraid to sound like they are whining. People are afraid if they share too much about the awful abyss that is autoimmune disease, at least too much at once, others will think they are attention-seeking, making it up, or that they are just being weak...but I am strong, I am brave, I am a fucking survivor and this shit sucks.

You are so fucking brave and strong too!

You deserve to know you are not alone, so I am going to try to write down every creak and every pain and every weird symptom so that you know this shit is real. It is unbearable. It matters. You aren't the only one.

I see you. I feel you. I believe you.

The classic symptoms of dermatomyositis are[23] (most of which I have the majority of the time):

*Gottron's papules or sign on the fingers and knuckles, elbows or knees, often split open into deep fissures that will split open and bleed by merely catching on a loose thread in a pocket or the pressure of opening a door

*Purple, lacy rash called the heliotrope rash on the face and eyes (including the more well-known butterfly rash), shoulders and chest (v-sign), neck (shawl), and thighs and upper legs (holster rash), and lower abdomen.

* Periungual telangiectasias—Nail fold and capillary changes on and in the skin leading up to cuticles which causes them to be painful and ragged.

*Diffuse itching and burning under the skin.

*Other skin lesions.

*Scalp involvement in advanced or untreated disease.

*Photosensitivity (even to fluorescent lights as well as the sun).

*Diffuse muscle weakness and pain.

*Calcifications in my breasts and armpits

*Trouble swallowing and voice changes

*GI involvement

*Symmetrical, proximal (hips, torso, and shoulder) muscle weakness.

*Difficulty standing from a seated position or from the floor

*Foot drop

*Fatigue

*Nerve damage

*Raynaud's syndrome often accompanies myositis

and more...

In addition, due to the normal, dermatomyositis-caused prolonged attack on my body, I have endured additional symptoms and results of dermatomyositis and its treatments. It feels unrelenting. It is impossible to list every single symptom and event, but if you bear with me, I will try to give a snapshot of the ones that have plagued me or have left the biggest impressions.

It is hard, no it's distressing, to list these. It's not because I'm a wilting flower, it's because of the constancy. It is because of the feeling of being locked-in, like one of those nightmares I described above. It is because even as a writer, there are not enough words to adequately tell you, dear reader, the hell in which I live, when I just pray for one day to be "okay." One moment in which I can walk hand-in-hand with my husband where I do not have to be aware of all the cracks in the sidewalk, so my toe doesn't catch, causing me to fall and break my nose and bust out my front tooth like on our honeymoon; or just scrape up my arms and hands like recently. I want just one afternoon with my kids when I can let myself be completely free and enjoy them without a muscle tremor here, or a nudge of pain there, or a stomach gurgle, or a pot I can't lift, or a vegetable I can't cut, or a word I can't remember.

I am forty-seven years old, but my wonderful family carries me through life as if I am eighty years old. Otherwise, I would miss out on all the big moments! In the best way possible they make me feel like a carefully tended fragile flower but also cherished, admired, and trusted. They make accommodations they shouldn't have to, to keep me included. Without their patience and ability to take things slower, to take the longer route, to take breaks, to point out the seating as soon as we enter a space, to call ahead for the easier options, I would miss out on their lives.

I actually did stay home for a long time until we figured out how to make excursions work for me. It was hard. It was alienating. It felt like I didn't have a place in their lives; not even as observer. I only got to see photos and hear stories. I missed seeing their adventures in kayaking, playing at the St. Louis City Museum (a playground for all ages), sledding in the park, hiking in the woods, walking in the parks and zoos, swimming at the pool, attending birthday parties for friends, and so much more. But after years of feeling left out, we learned that with a cane or rollator, at first, and then if taken in small doses, with breaks or naps in between I don't have to miss out on as much. I started being able to go back to being along for the ride, even with the accommodations in place.

I have lost *so many* friends due to canceled lunches from being too ill or tired. I couldn't drive at night for years due to all my eye surgeries, so I couldn't meet up for dinners or drinks (not that I can drink much anyway because of medications and low tolerance). I have lost friends due to "not asking for help" (sorry you can't bathe me!). I have lost friends for being too sad or sick all the time (sorry my disease is a buzz kill). I know I am not alone in this, others I know with chronic illness talk about how isolating illness is, how even family members don't listen or understand how all-encompassing it is. We aren't making it up, and we aren't exaggerating. That's part of why I am letting it all hang out here. I am doing it so you know you aren't alone in this unrelenting, tiring, tireless bullshit that wears you down, it chews you up and spits you out and then repeats the whole process. Honestly, if anyone thinks you are making it up, well they aren't really listening to you, are they?

Often, when I seem "good," I'm probably faking it so that I can have some semblance of a life. In a fit of emotional pain and rage against my illness, Sage once accused me of faking being sick. She was about eleven or twelve years old, and we had just gotten home from her skating session (I talk a lot about skating as it was one of the only reasons I left the house without Scott for many years to conserve my energy). She noted that I seemed incongruently happy when I watched her skate or talked to other parents at the rink but when we returned home, I collapsed and napped while she did her independent homeschool work after I taught her the lessons. She also noted that she felt I took advantage of her dad, my husband, as he did (and still does) most of the housework but I was this bubbly person she didn't recognize when we were out.

I told her she had it backwards. I was faking being well! I was using all my energy and strength to be able to be part of her life, to have friends in person, outside the house; often napping in the car when she had her coach(es) on the ice with her or knowing other adults were present so she was safe. While I relished and enjoyed the interactions, I was completely depleted when we got home. There were days it took all I had to muster the strength to drive home, and maybe there were days I shouldn't have driven home, and sometimes even having to call for someone to come get us.

As for daddy doing all the housework, despite his long work hours; by the time he got home and I had cooked dinner, after taking her to the rink, doing homeschool with her, even with naps, I had nothing left...sometimes having difficulty even sitting up for the entire meal.

Small exertions that look like nothing to others cause me bone wrenching pain, fatigue that feels like molasses in my veins or 100-pound weights attached to each joint and muscle, and tiredness that is distinguishable from fatigue yet indescribable (people who have experienced it know what I am talking about, you cannot keep your eyes open no matter what, and it is utter hell on earth). I know my sweet little one didn't mean to hurt me more, on top of my body's betrayal, but knowing that even she saw me differently than what was really happening made it so much worse. It has become an involuntary refrain that plays over and over in my head and makes me question, even more than before, "am I faking this?", when new outrageous symptoms appear.

It's even hard when people tell me I don't look sick. Like, seriously, what am I supposed to say to that? Thanks? It is really hard when it feels so invalidating. I am doing everything I can to stay upright, but you, stranger, or friend don't think I look sick? Or how about the time someone told me that my rash looked terrible when it was actually in a decent phase. Why do people feel the need to comment? How about a simple, "Hi, nice to see you?" Sometimes even, in a protracted and drawn out voice, "Ohhh how are you feeeeeling?" is a loaded and difficult question. Many people ask that, but don't even stick around for more than the typical, "I'm okay," answer.

One of the kindest and most empathetic and things anyone says to me about my health is from Sage's coach, Chris. He doesn't blithely ask, "How are you?" (Which, again, isn't a measure of anything for me and is an offhanded question often people ask without waiting for an answer anyway.)

When I am strong enough to go to the rink to watch her skate, he always says some version of, "I am so glad to see you are up to being here today. I know it takes a lot so thank you for being here to encourage Sage, I appreciate your efforts." How lovely. No assumption that my disease disappeared, no asking me to quantify my pain, no off-handed, "how are you?," no assessment of me by his untrained and uninvited eye. It is a recognition of how sick I am, how hard I work to come, and how important being there is for both Sage and me.

What a great example of empathy, love, and support! We are lucky to have him in her life!

———

NOW, JUST TO BE AS thoroughly grotesque as humanly possible, I'm going to list as many of the symptoms and side effects I can think of that I have encountered as well as ones my friends have told me about. I do this to expose the yuck, give voice to the voiceless, and demystify the unrelenting disease processes because we aren't faking being sick. We are doing our best to live through illness, to find the best, but sometimes this shit just sucks.

Being sick sucks. The autoimmune abyss is endless and daunting. It feels like it will swallow you whole and no one will even know you were there. Sometimes, just when you think you've had a couple of good days, a bad, bad day pops up to remind you that your illness is always there. We fake being well, because the alternative is to give up, to crawl into bed, curl up into a ball and wait for the end. It doesn't work. I've tried.

Here we go…

First, I'll attempt to list my other diagnoses and symptoms on top of and concurrent with dermatomyositis:

*fibromyalgia

*autoimmune urticaria (chronic hives)

*dysautonomia

*painful DM-related calcifications in my armpits and breasts *neuropathy

*chronic shingles

*chronic migraines

*celiac plus additional food sensitivities

*pityriasis amiantacea—the technical term for my scalp's hard, nail-like lesions

*incongruent distal muscle weakness (hands and feet)

*osteopenia (thinning bones)

*chronic and multiple retinal detachments in both eyes and associated complications starting at 32, including repeated posterior vitreous detachments, retinal hemorrhages, macular puckers, and getting cataracts at 36 years old — which may have also been contributed to from shingles

*alternating anemia, leukopenia, and neutropenia from chronic immune suppression

*multiple miscarriages

*a hysterectomy at 32 resulting from years of painful and hemorrhaging periods as well as the miscarriages

*endometriosis and ovarian cysts

*adrenal impairment

*Irritable bowel syndrome

Plus, once someone is taking immune suppressant drugs, there are many other risks that come into play. Immune suppression makes a person more susceptible to infection, difficulty in healing from wounds or surgeries.

My back usually feels like it's breaking in half from a combination of the neuropathy, muscle spasms, tendons and ligaments contracting, and weakness that causes horrible posture. This is worse if I overexert, even a little.

I am always blinking away floaters because of all my eye surgeries. Whether the blood floaters are translucent or obstructive they are distracting. There is large jellyfish floater that's part of a current posterior vitreous detachment that we can't take out because my eyes are too unstable from too many past surgeries.

I have chronic shingles even though I've had the vaccine **and** I take Valtrex every day to prevent them.

I have scalp involvement that spans anywhere from large dry itchy flakes, to blistering and bleeding lesions, to huge crusty plaques that feel like fingernails or porcupine needles growing out of my scalp (pityriasis amiantacea). I have bald patches. I shed skin like a reptile. I have itching pain that cuts so deep it causes my skull to ache and burn. I have red, purple, and silver splotches on my temples, face, scalp, and ears that hurt but are also embarrassing and gross even ME out.

As I mentioned before, I look fairly "normal" unless you watch me move or look at me closely. Unfortunately, my rash is quite visible close up and I have lost a large portion of my hair. In fact, as much as people like to assess my rash, it should be a work of art and I should be getting paid residuals.

I am always bleeding or bruised, somewhere.

I have overgrown cuticles that feel like sharp fingernails and catch, pop, and break; bleeding dark flowing blood that shouldn't come from such a small skin cut.

I have had hereditary ingrown toenails since I was a kid, but as my Dermatomyositis and resultant Raynaud's have both worsened and the combination of lack of blood flow and overgrowth of cuticles have increased, I now have them on every toe. Pedicures do not help. I've had the surgery on my big toes multiple times. The ingrown nails that were partially "removed" grew back, but worse. Also, with immune suppression, my toes get infected easily (I will give gory details on many things, but all I'll say here is puss. Lots of puss. Because puss...it is gross.). I tried to manage them with frequent pedicures, but they aren't effective long-term. I soak my feet and do a lot of self-care on my cuticles and trimming my nails, but I finally saw a podiatrist (remember the insurance company tried to deny it?) to address a couple of the infected ones and we decided that the best plan was to see him for individual toes as they flare up. He said he would cut them back but as I have not had success with the conventional treatment, and there is a risk for infection, he is hesitant to repeat it. Again, I am left to deal with something in an ongoing fashion, that other people can get fixed, albeit painfully, but my DM is making the toes more of an issue than normal. On top of it, now I, **again,** have to worry about dealing with insurance about the damn visits.

My IBS includes firehose diarrhea with searing and tearing pain. It is exacerbated by medications and has led to dehydration.

I have migraines that last days and make the light coming under a closed door feel like knives.

I have experienced mental status changes, like mentioned earlier with both steroids and Jak inhibitors.

I get rashes, vomiting, fevers, migraines, dizziness, diarrhea, weakness, foggy vision, swollen body parts, anxiety, mouth sores, shingles, throat closing thrush, and so many more examples of side effects from other medications.

There is never a minute when I am awake that one part of my body isn't betraying me, and it gets old. No matter how wonderful Scott is, it is hard to believe anyone around me truly understands how incessant it is.

I'm supposed to just live with this. I'm supposed to just be like this and everyone else goes along with their day, but I feel stupid that sometimes I can't see "right" out of one eye. I got my eyes tested and told the doctor about the days they don't focus. I asked if two scripts would help. He said, "no, that's just inflammation inhibiting focus." In other words, *just accept there will be days you cannot fucking see.*

Sometimes I can't recognize my own husband when I come out of a public bathroom in certain lighting so he always stands in a pre-agreed upon place so I can find him! I can't find Sage in a crowd, because I am unable to scan faces and on really bad eye days, I can't even pick her out on the ice rink, the place she is at every day, because the light enters my eyes weirdly and I just can't make her out. This happened once when she was little, and I spent an *eternity* thinking Sage had been kidnapped. Five minutes into my *eternal* freak out, I asked a friend for help finding her...the friend pointed out that she was working quietly on a spin technique in the back corner of the ice. The lighting and my eyes had made it so I just couldn't focus well enough to differentiate her from the rest of the skaters because everything was hooded and darkened, and her face was blurred like I was looking through water. That still happens to me now; but I know it will eventually pass. Seriously, I have to accept that I will have time periods of unfixable sight.

At least once a day a foot goes to sleep but it doesn't really go to sleep. I have shooting electrical shocks that feel like it is on fire. Or I stand up and the cramp is so bad in my foot that I can't flatten it and it is unrelenting and over and over and over and on and on and on.

I'm a screaming broken record.

And because I've set myself up as the person who is always in a good mood, I usually try to do all of this with a fucking smile on my face. But I've started to wonder if some of that is actually a coping mechanism bordering on a little bit of denial rather than always "looking on the bright side"? I mean, if you have scalding skin, electrical shocks, feet and legs that go out from under you at any moment how happy can you really be, all the time? I've come to understand that being happy and finding my *moments of divinity* are good goals, but I don't have to do it all the time. I can be fucking pissed as much as I want. I can be crabby. I can be angry. I don't owe anyone a smile.

Knowing that I'm costing a fortune to keep comfortable to stop some pain and keep alive is sometimes overwhelming. I question if that is too much or if it may become so in the future. I cannot tell you how many times I have cried to my best friend about the vulnerability I feel over money. Not that I think Scott will leave me, but I never pictured myself being dependent on another person to this extent.

It isn't easy to watch my medical bills rise and nonexistent savings continue to not exist. I'm lucky. Scott has an amazing job with a great salary. I feel immense gratitude for our financial situation, because I am acutely aware that had it not been for him, I would have nothing. I legitimately cannot work; I do not come from a family that would be able to support me if I were alone and if I didn't have Scott I do not know how my health situation would be today.

None of this feels good. Yet I am grateful. I realize that I am safe and that many people with chronic illness do not enjoy the security that I do, they do not have the insurance I have, flawed as it is, and they do not enjoy the emotional support I do nor the license to voice their fears, feelings, and physical woes as I do.

For eight long years I fought for my disability and appealed against unfair denials. I was finally approved this fall after years of demoralizing, disgusting, degrading, disrespectful, and inappropriate questions at my hearings where my ethics and honesty were called into question despite having thousands of pages (I think my lawyer said nearly 10,000) of medical records documenting the severity of my disease and letters from three doctors plus the testimony of two vocational rehab specialists and an independent doctor all saying I would not be able to hold down a job of any kind. As hard as all of that was to endure, it is an immense relief to finally have this behind us.

THIS is the problem with silencing sick people. **We all** have the *right* and the *need* to be heard. **We all** *deserve* to be supported. We deserve to have the financial security of insurance, disability payments, knowing we can get out medicine, eat, have a roof over our heads, at minimum have our needs met (although I don't know how that is all we should strive for as humans).

It is a human right to have acceptable, adequate healthcare.[24] The last thing a sick person should be worried about is paying for medicine, yet that is often the first thing we have to think about when the doctor orders any new medication, "Will the insurance company deny it?" and/or "How long will the appeals take to get the insurance approval?" and "What will my out-of-pocket-cost be?" because no matter how much money you/your household makes, if you hit your deductible in the first couple of months every year, and the out-of-pocket max in fourth or fifth month, over the years that can add up to an enormous amount of money.

Sage asked us how much money we spend on my healthcare. Let me start with the caveat that I am extremely fortunate that I have even been able to pay what we have. I owe my life to my husband's career and ability to pay for care. Not a day goes by that I do not feel and express gratitude for the fact that I have the best healthcare I could have under this flawed system. But that doesn't mean that that great health insurance doesn't still make me suffer indignities.

We estimated that, from 2005-2022, if we spent at least an average deductible/out-of-pocket-max of $4000-5000/year, sometimes more and sometimes less depending on the year and his employer's plan. Taking seventeen years times $5000 equals approximately $85,000 in copays, medications, and other direct payments to medical providers to keep me alive. This is a wholly cautious number because I believe the $5000 to be a low average over those seventeen years.

We could count the number of extraneous treatments we have tried that were not covered by insurance. We could add in travel expenses from St. Louis to Kansas City when I traveled to KU every couple of months for specialists, as well as other travel to other specialists. We could add in the extra money we spend on specialized food due to my terribly sensitive stomach (healthy food is not cost-effective nor is it widely available and we should change that in this country). We also could go further to figure in my lost wages as an attorney.

I am not sitting at home for fun. Anyone who thinks that sitting home when you had dreams of working in human rights to better the world has no idea the anguish of watching your dreams die — one symptom, one rash, one shot, one pill, one infusion, and one hospital visit at a time. I am fighting for my life and taking the most horrible drugs to do so, even though they do terrible things, hoping their good outweighs the bad. (Some do and some don't.) I cannot work. There is no job on the planet that would allow for the number of absences, naps, doctor appointments, treatments, etc., that I need to survive; much less missing the sick days I would take for disease symptoms.

Finally, many people with autoimmune disease develop cardiovascular and lung involvement. Malignancy is highly indicated in myositis (and other autoimmune diseases),[25] especially in the first few years of myositis.[26]

I recently read about diseases that wildly fluctuate being described as "dynamic."[27]

So the next time someone insinuates that you can't be "that sick" or they "saw you go for a walk with your family so how can you be sick today?", have them read this chapter. I believe you. They should too!

Chapter 9
Disability Porn

"U + Ur Hand," by P!nk

***I**'m writing this chapter a little differently. I hope patients feel comfortable sharing it with others.*

How can I say this delicately, but clearly enough so non-sick people will understand it? We (people with chronic illness and people with disabilities) are not here to entertain you and we are certainly not here to make you feel better about yourselves by throwing a couple dollars at a quick GoFundMe here and there or by wearing a sticker! (In writing this paragraph I realize I have also heard this complaint from my friends in other marginalized populations, so I do not think we are alone in this.)

Granted, I mostly have an invisible disability, and my time using a walker and a cane is intermittent and transient. Although I am "permanently disabled," meaning I will never get better, and will never be able to work a full-time job again...either way, I do not have the experiences of all people with all illnesses and disabilities, so I cannot speak to the full experience of people living in different situations. It is completely up to the individual how much they do or do not move into the public view. I do know, however, that when I hear certain things my blood boils and I wonder where real compassion has gone. P!nk's song just plays over and over in my head.

I realize that as long as the person who has the disease or disability controls the narrative and discussion that is one thing, but as soon as someone else, often the media, starts to talk for us, then it becomes about clicks, likes, and garnering "sympathy" for a cause instead of spreading awareness.

Please allow me a moment to give credit where it is due. I learned about the importance of true allyship a couple of years ago in learning and reading about the Anti-Racism conversation.[28] A universal truth we could all use reminding of (which these teachers made very clear) is when you count someone as your equal, your behavior shows that. The difference, as I understood it, is first we have to confront our biases. Then, allyship means taking the lead from the person or persons being affected by the unfair treatment, injustice, or discrimination as opposed to imposing your agenda on them and taking the spotlight to look like a good person. (This is a poignant parallel to remember that people with Black and Brown skin are under-represented in all the medical journals and have to fight harder to be taken seriously than their white counterparts.)[29]

When I learned that about allyship with anti-racism, it helped me to put into words something that had bothered me for a long time about how people with illness are treated. Often "caring about" disease and disability are touted as symbolic of how helpful a charity is, or how well-meaning a celebrity is, or how much a sports team cares about community.

Some people with illness do choose to be the face of a disease. That's 100% their choice to spread awareness, and I applaud them! I mean, I write about and talk about being sick all the time, I can hardly complain when people ask me about my illness! My problem is when a line is crossed from the person spreading awareness and an organization using them to make others feel warm and fuzzy, I'm not sure how clear that line is. I know it is up to the person who is in the public eye, first and foremost, but I also think we as a community of people coping with illness have an opportunity to demand we are treated with respect and dignity and that the people asking for us to show our faces are doing so in the spirit of allyship not just for warm fuzzies.

But really, isn't the truth that the more you do to help others without doing it for recognition or accolades, the more altruistic it is?[30]

I think true allies write letters to representatives in congress asking for better funding for rare diseases, or disability access, or for proper healthcare. This would be far better than standing on a stage talking about how great they are at helping people who are disabled or sick but are "so brave" and have "overcome so much" (excuse me while I gag at the patronizing nature of such speeches).

Additionally, on the same lines, VOTE! Vote to make healthcare more affordable so your friends with chronic illnesses and disabilities aren't stressing about paying for their medications. People literally die because they can't afford their medications and/or insurance companies deny them.[31] Where is your allyship then? Where are your warm fuzzies then?

In my opinion, another, more personal way to help is to see if you can bring your friend dinner or offer to give your friend rides to the doctor if they are struggling with fatigue or stop by the grocery store when they are unable to leave the house. These would be delicate conversations, of course, and would need to be handled with care, possibly started with "I know you have said you are having a rough time, is there anything I can do to lighten your load? I would love to bring a home cooked dinner for your family." Or, "I've noticed you mentioned it is difficult to go to the grocery store recently, would a ride there help ease your fatigue?" Or "Would it be helpful for me to pick up a few things on my way home from work?" Always acknowledging their words about the struggle before making an offer is helpful so they know you aren't coming at them with pity but approaching them with empathy and love. I have always felt more cared for when friends approach me this way rather than the "why don't you do [xyz] anymore?" or "Why won't you let me help you?"

An even more global, way to help, rather than patronize, is to donate money to patient-led initiatives who know what the patients need and know how to properly put the time and money to the best use to advocate for patients' real needs. They know how to contact the stakeholders who have the power to change our lives, and they have the language and experience to convey the seriousness of our conditions, from firsthand knowledge. That's why I think patient-led initiatives are so much more successful through organizations like Myositis Support and Understanding and International Foundation for Autoimmune & Autoinflammatory Arthritis because they have patients talking about their experiences and not being hijacked by non-patients speaking for us.

I'll try to break it down gently, there is a fine line to expressing gratitude for someone you knows illness being in remission, or their progress in getting "stronger" which is relative anyway, and there is even value in expressing to someone how happy you are for them having a good day...but I am an outspoken advocate for people with chronic illness, invisible diseases, autoimmune and myositis specifically and I have to tell you I am so tired of hearing about how inspiring I am. How brave I am. What a fighter I am.

I am not brave. I don't have a choice! I would not be here if I didn't buck up and do what the fucking doctors say. Even though it is probably said with all good intentions, it sometimes feels demeaning. The most demeaning ones are the news stories, in my opinion. It is probably the media stories of someone who "triumphs" over their illness. Guess what, we triumph every fucking day by existing and those same people making a big deal about the triumphs are also running us over in the aisles at the store, blocking the disabled parking spots when the pick their kids up at the gym, they are scoffing at us when we take a few extra minutes to order food because we need to make sure the order is safe for our allergies and sensitivities.

One of my biggest regrets is worrying if TMT was misinterpreted by the non-sick world as disability porn. I've spent the last few years being afraid that I contributed to it by writing a book about how you can be happy while you're sick and giving license to those who want to minimize our experiences. I wrote it to inspire *US* to find the positives of *OUR* experiences, but in recent years I have seen so much belittling for the illness experience and would hate that my words could be used to further that cause. I absolutely abhor that anyone could look at that type of attitude say, "Oh that's so inspiring" and then they expect the same from other people.

We are all at different places and not everyone is ready to bright-side this shit, hell, we aren't even all always ready to bright-side from one day to the next! There's a difference between wanting to inspire other people who are sick, and that goal being bastardized into healthy or able-bodied people using disability as inspiration, which, in my opinion is code for a lack of respect for what we actually go through.

I don't really know if I can explain this any better, except the next time you see a sick person, treat them like you'd want to be treated. If they ask for help and you are able then do that, if they ask to be treated like "just one of the group," do that. Let their actions, boundaries, and desires guide you, just like you would with any other friend.

Chapter 10
Getting Over Vanity Means Getting Creative;

TMI Coming Your Way!

"About Damn Time," by Lizzo (Watch her official video if you can)

I've had to get over so much of my vanity and pride in favor of taking better care of myself. I am petrified of stinking, looking greasy, wearing clothes that look dirty, etc.

I hate that I shed so much hair and skin that I leave my DNA on my clothes and everywhere I go. I try to avoid dark shirts when I can so that I don't have that trademark "snow" visible on my shoulders. I have hard, bleeding, ragged cuticles. I bleed from skin ulcers spontaneously. I have fish-like scales that feel like fingernails on my scalp, and I sometimes have snot drip from my nose even without knowing it is coming out (thank you nerve damage!).

I have come up with many creative ways to manage things that would otherwise be demoralizing; but that doesn't mean I always feel good about them, and it really doesn't make the reality of them less disconcerting.

I'm putting my own embarrassment front and center to share these situations because I want you to know it's okay; and to be fair, I am not truly ashamed of these things anymore. I have a supportive husband and we have made adaptations in this regard to help me feel as clean and "put together" as I can. In the end the only person's opinion I really care about is Scott's.

When you are sick, hygiene sucks. I don't mean that **your** hygiene sucks. I mean **taking care of** hygiene sucks.

For instance, because of fatigue, I only shower every couple of days; otherwise, I use up all my energy for the remainder of the day. In fact, most of the time, after a shower I need to lie down for a few minutes to recharge before I can go on with my day (I hear this from so many of my friends with chronic illness and chronic pain). Plus, my skin gets angrier and drier the more I shower (if you can believe that is possible!).

I have digestive issues (IBS with diarrhea), hemorrhoids, past hemorrhoid surgery, and a rectocele (my rectum folds in half, sideways, when I poop instead of scrunching straight down) so I have anal leakage of the poop that is never fully expelled. It is uncomfortable when I try to defecate, and it is itchy and self-conscious to worry that I may smell sometimes. Although this makes cleanliness even more crucial; even as showering daily is out of the question. We have also found that installing a fairly inexpensive bidet in our bathroom has helped immensely. I also use, as one friend calls them, "bougie," sensitive baby wipes to clean my booty and my body, like a sponge bath, daily. Wash cloths would probably accomplish the same goal if that is your preference, and I use a wash cloth in the shower, of course, but I find carrying baby wipes with me everywhere makes me feel safe and clean so my butt is always baby fresh.

Even more than the limited showers, I only wash my hair twice a week. Thankfully, it helps my scalp to wash my hair less. I kept my hair short for years but grew it out thinking a ponytail would be easier to manage and cover up my bald spots. A while ago, I decided to cut it back off. Not only does the shorter, oddly, fuller style cover up my sores and bald spots, it has helped my scalp pain, slightly, not to have it in a ponytail. The "finger nails" growing out of my scalp (pityriasis amiantacea) are still there, but not as irritated. I didn't realize how much pulling it back was putting pressure on those plaques and stressing my scalp out more. It hasn't stopped any of the problems, but it has decreased the stress on my little 'ole noggin.

I have also recently realized that it is helping even more to rinse it many days and only use shampoo every other wash. I don't dry my hair, I towel fluff it, comb it, and walk away. The less I touch it the better.

On the topic of other hair, I don't shave! Legs, armpits, pubic area, nothing... I stopped about 10 years ago. I found that shaving aggravated the internal "fire ant" burning pain in my legs and it intensified the external sores. I occasionally trim my armpit hair when it gets too long and starts to itch, I've nearly lost all my pubic hair, and the hair on my legs appears to have stopped growing and is way softer. I have always questioned the patriarchal social construct that exclusively tells women to shave their legs, anyway, so it was a nice change to stop shaving my legs! Now I wonder why I spent so much time and energy on it to begin with.

Next, oral hygiene. I have some wretched dry mouth from my medications and from my disease. I just had my semi-annual dental appointment. My dental report was very good. I had very little plaque, almost no tartar, and no concerns with my gums; the only concern is that my jaw is slipping to the side, so I have to go to the jaw orthopedic to have it checked to be sure there is no jaw muscle deterioration.

But pertaining to mouth health, they even complimented me on my stellar flossing. I have some confessions to make. I've never flossed a day in my life! (Not that I am recommending not flossing, I'm just telling my truth.)

I gag badly and have since I was a kid. I have problems with my jaw and cannot open my mouth widely enough to floss (even the hygienist has trouble with flossing the back teeth). I only brush my teeth once a day in the morning because I cannot open my mouth wide enough to brush them at night due to the jaw fatigue and gagging.

During the worst part of the pandemic when I was not comfortable going to the dentist for nearly 20 months, I got a Waterpik toothbrush and used the hell out of it. I use the vibrating brush carefully on all sides of each tooth and then go back and use the Waterpik flossing function the same way. When I went for my first cleaning after I was vaccinated, they said they couldn't tell it had been as long as it had since my last professional cleaning, yay for technology!

This next topic is taboo and hard to talk about. I'll be really honest. My weight has fluctuated between 125 and about 180 in the twenty-eight years I have been sick. I am somewhere between 5'2 and 5'3 depending on the day and how I am feeling (did you know that affects your height?). That means I have technically been both under-nourished and obese. This isn't because I can't control my own eating, it is because my medicines cause weird, rapid gains and losses; without much change in my diet. And I don't have any elasticity to accommodate the weight changes so I have weird looking skin, especially in my abdomen and neck. I have had some muscle loss throughout the years, so my skin hangs funny in places and fat deposits end up in weird places with hollow spots next to them.

Here are the specifics. My most common weight over the years has probably been between 150-160; but it isn't comfortable at my height with no muscles of which to speak. My most comfortable weight, to physically carry around and look in the mirror, was probably 135 (but I was having trouble getting food in my body, and my CBC showed it isn't my healthiest).

I'll admit, as body-positive as I try to be, I am personally losing the battle on this. I would prefer to be smaller. I am short. I have a small frame, big boobs, and small bones. My skin elasticity is gone, I have droopy skin when I lose weight and stretched out, shiny, busting-open skin when I gain it. I can move better when I am smaller. I like my face better without the steroid and inflammation induced swollen moon face. I liked wearing smaller clothes and not having rolls. But I have also recently been reminding myself that I am forty-seven, happily married, and alive. I wrote a whole chapter in TMT on body image, so it is clearly an ongoing issue for me. I try to remember that hating my body's look is definitely not going to help it.

I know and fully believe — on the outside — that what matters is that I am alive and that I can function. I know my husband loves me for who I am, not how I look. But it is a daily struggle. I want my body to cooperate and not gain weight for no reason. I have built up a little more muscle than I had in the past, right now, so I am trying to keep that at the forefront of my mind, but damn, it is hard.

Since this can be one of the hardest parts of chronic illness for many people, because it affects us on the outside, but also psychologically, I want to mention another song that I love to listen to, *Scars to Your Beautiful* by Alessia Cara. She wrote it about some personal health struggles and as she "promotes a message of self-acceptance that challenges the beautify standards we see every day."[32]

Just know, if you are struggling with any of this too, you are not alone. Letting go of some of the image in your head of what you looked like in the past doesn't change who you are. It is just adjusting to *what is*.

But, yeah, it still fucking sucks, because say it with me: **Being Sick Sucks**.

Chapter 11
"So No One Told You Life Was Gonna Be This Way"

———

In Memory of Matthew Perry 1969-2023

"I'll Be There for You (Friend's Theme)," by The Rembrandts

*N*ote: *I wrote this chapter in November of 2022. I am editing it in November of 2023, a couple of weeks after his sudden passing. I am inordinately and irrationally sad that I cannot send a book to him and tell him about how much his book helped me. On one hand I want to be realistic and say he probably would not have seen it anyway, but somehow, I think he would have, based on the accounts of the kind of person he was. Anyway, this chapter is dedicated to Matthew Perry a great actor, and from all accounts, an even better human.*

I read *Friends, Lovers, and the Big Terrible Thing: A Memoir,*[33] by Matthew Perry in an exceedingly short period for the serious subject matter contained therein because I couldn't put it down. I was struck by how relentless addiction is and how similar Perry's words about his struggle with addiction and mental health were to my struggle with autoimmune disease.

Perry's story burrowed into my soul. The theme song from friends played in a continuous loop in my head as I read his book as he talked about the people who stuck it out with him. The eponymous song's refrain, "I'll Be There for You..." rang through as a theme. I couldn't help but compare it to how I have people in my life who are always here for me.

Perry talked about addiction as if it is a medical condition. Guess what? It is![34] Perry talked about mental health as if it is a medical condition. Guess what? It is![35]

His book brought me to thinking about the people I know who deal with addiction and/or mental illness. I thought about how they are mistreated by the medical community in the same way people with chronic illness and autoimmune disease are. I also thought about how people with autoimmune disease are dismissed by the medical establishment as being mentally ill and drug seeking as if minimizing physical symptoms as mental illness makes us less important.

But, newsflash, mental illness is not a scarlet letter. It shouldn't be used as a divisive way to prevent care for autoimmune disease, chronic pain, chronic illness, or anything else the doctors do not understand. And it sure as hell should not be seen as a sword or shield that is used to make patients with any condition feel they are "making it up" or "just here for drugs" because that serves to minimize the experiences of people with mental illness and addiction. This in turn minimizes the experience of the person with autoimmune disease, chronic pain, etc. Rinse and repeat. It is a vicious cycle of nothingness that **helps no one and hurts everyone**. In a word, it is just vicious.

As I read Perry's book, I realized that the medical establishment will do anything they can to dismiss and belittle that which they don't understand. If Perry, who had seemingly unlimited money and attended many rehabs and had multiple procedures, interventions, etc., continued to struggle for years while putting on a happy face...I don't think it means we have no hope, I think it means we need to overhaul the system and look at how we treat our bodies. We need to look at how to medical system mistreats people with chronic conditions of all kinds. We need to get honest about medical abuse and neglect.

It is time for it to stop.

Perry's book is one such way to open the eyes of the medical community, every medical professional should be required to read it. He was funny and engaging and real. He told a tragic story of pain and multiple brushes with death; as well as his feelings of invincibility and his own staring into the abyss of addiction and feeling alone even when surrounded by many (millions in his case).

Doctors of all specialties could learn from him to be more compassionate, to take the time to understand how addiction and mental illness affect every aspect of life, and to treat the whole person (not just what many see as character flaws) — because again, they are not.

My books are another way to educate medical personnel. People living without chronic illness, especially without autoimmune disease, should be required to read the real-life stories of those of us living them every day. Doctors of all specialties could learn from me, and people like me, to be more compassionate, to take the time to understand how chronic illnesses affect every aspect of life, and to treat the whole person (not just what many see as character flaws) — because again, they are not. We are not making this shit up. It is okay to cry, and that doesn't make us out of touch with reality, it means we know how bad it is...because...Being Sick Sucks.

Whether the person is there with one chronic illness or many chronic illnesses, it doesn't matter. Whether the person is there with addiction, or mental illness, or both; or even, all of the above also doesn't matter. We are not in the office to annoy the doctor. We are not there for "attention-seeking." We are there for the medical person's undivided *medical* attention, care, and unbiased assistance. We are not there because we want to be, we are there because we have to be if we want to be **here, as in *alive*!**

Something Perry said hit me strongly because I read it shortly after the second time a Jak-inhibitor medication gave me suicidal ideation thoughts. It was as if he said something he had plucked directly from my mind, so I am passing it on to you in the hope it helps someone:

Perry said, "So, there I was, living in a Malibu sober living house on 8 milligrams of Suboxone. Though it's a solid detox drug — the best — as I've said over and over, it is the hardest drug on the planet to get off. In fact, it made me suicidal to come off it. That's not quite accurate—I had suicidal feelings, but I also knew it was just the medicine, so I wasn't actually suicidal, if you follow."[36]

He, like me, knew the suicidal thoughts were not his own. I hope if you ever have this low, dangerous, horrible thought, yourself, you will be able to see it for what it is, as he did, and as I did too, as an outside, transient thought that someone can help you with. That is not to cause any shame or guilt. It is a strong and terribly real thought, but hopefully being equipped with the information is helpful to hold on long enough to ask for help.

It is this perspective of knowing the thought wasn't my own (and subsequently calling my husband and best friend the first time; and being able to articulate the thought immediately the second time a year later) that kept me from acting on the thought. It felt implanted or outside of me but still inside my head. If this happens at any time, please call for help. I am listing some resources in the endnotes.[37]

I think the main thing I took away from reading this book was that just like my peers and I don't feel like we are taken seriously enough, I think mental health and addiction are similarly rebuffed in the medical field. I think it is time that that stops for all of us.

Thank you, Matthew Perry, wherever you are, for having exposed your scariest times for us to see, absorb, mourn for, and hopefully learn and grow from. We are better for you having shared your struggles with us and we are left worse for your loss. I truly hope you are at peace and send my condolences to your family.

Chapter 12
Immune Suppression in a Pandemic

—

"No One is Alone," from Into the Woods

by Anna Kendrick, James Corden Lilla Crawford, Daniel Huttlestone

COVID's rampant circling of the globe showed how un-alone we are and our interconnectedness. I think we failed as humans. It exposed the lack of compassion for others. I can't tell you how many times I heard "the people who are vulnerable and die from COVID were going to die anyway" while my doctors were telling me that I would likely not survive COVID (prior to vaccination); except I was not in immediate danger of dying from dermatomyositis unless I got COVID. This was even said by people I knew personally.

My family lived in near complete isolation for over 6-8 months. Our son Rickey and his fiancé Tiffany started to bring us groceries after we saw the amount of money it was costing in delivery fees. Scott would spend hours wiping every item off before bringing it into the house. For the first couple of weeks, we were instructed to get our medications delivered early so they could sit in the garage a week or so before bringing them into the house. There was no information about if it could live on the individual pills and you couldn't wash pills!

My brother would visit us outside, bringing his two small kids, around four and seven years old at the time, to our house. We would sit in the driveway, while they played in the yard, and talk. For a long time, we sat twenty feet apart because we didn't know anything about the transmissibility of the virus, then as we knew more we gradually sat closer, but never closer than ten feet apart unless masked. We once went for a walk at the park with them, masked, when the county first lifted the lock down. As much as I loved seeing them up close, I was so scared for days afterward that I would get COVID from my sweet innocent nephews. It was a nightmare. Thankfully, the boys were very sweet and my brother and the boys' mom did an excellent job of helping them understand why I couldn't hug them and play like normal. They were empathetic and cautious. It was wonderful when the day came that I could hug them both again.

For about 20-24 months we were completely masked and distanced while carefully trying to live in the new world, only starting to remove our masks carefully and for very short periods of time in the beginning of 2023. We masked long into 2023 except in small groups. Thankfully we are not doing so anymore. I know people who are still living in near complete isolation because they are high risk and not able to vaccinate or mask. They matter and they report that the isolation is unbearable at times.

We have received all the vaccines available to us, but the impact the pandemic had on our 17-year-old (fourteen at the beginning), and the time we lost with loved ones, including cherished loved ones who have since died — to protect me — is immeasurable.

We contracted COVID in January of 2022. Sage and Scott were only sick a couple of days, thanks to the vaccines and good immune systems. I was sick for nearly three weeks, with "mild to moderate symptoms" according to the official classification, but thanks to Paxlovid was able to stay home and was not "severe" even though it didn't feel "mild" or "moderate" at all at the time.

This poem I wrote (below) sums up my feelings about how we handled the pandemic. Each person's actions affect another.

———————————

COVID KILLED THE HUGGERS

By Emily A. Filmore

Pandemic precautions, Wiped down, six feet apart. A dangerous virus, hugging friends becomes a lost art.

Immune suppression, severe health conditions, age, medications, and other vulnerabilities. Exposures amount to more than a cold, rendering movement a severe liability.

Masks, sanitizers, vaccines, and great air purifiers help others return to a more normal life, still those of us living in grave danger, continue to face tremendous strife.

We've begged for consideration, we've asked for empathy. We've pleaded not to be discarded, but COVID attitudes'll go down in infamy.

Nearly seven million souls dead, worldwide, since March 2020, "Life moves on," it is said, and they claim we've "recovered." But have we? Look around! Compassion's expir'd. Affection is gone, COVID killed the huggers.

Chapter 13
Progress and the Inevitable Fall:
The Abyss Yawns On

"Slow it Down," by The Lumineers

Right as I was finishing this book, I fell down about four stairs at the bottom of a stairwell. It is my biggest fall in a while, although I have falls and near-misses every couple of weeks.

I don't know exactly how it happened, but I slipped from my "foot drop" and some flaw in the stairs (not at my house). I bump — bump — bumped down those last few steps on my ass. This is not the first time and won't be the last.

Part of the problem is I do not have a startle reflex anymore, so I don't react fast enough and try to catch myself. That's why I fall so easily, so often, and so hard. I have had the crown on my front tooth, and the lateral next to it, replaced a couple of times because I keep falling on my face. Yep, falling is expensive. I have an Apple Watch to alert my husband and 911 if I have a bad fall. I have had bad falls with my watch on, and it has only detected one, so it is no help! It didn't notice my fall down the stairs!

Anyway, the stairs netted me a bruised ass and legs, sore ankles (not sprained, just sore), and a sore, twisted back. ...plus an increasingly busted ego.

I was talking to Scott about it the next morning, while I was checking my body over for scrapes and bruises. I sobbed as I told him that I am tired of feeling like I am gaining ground but then finding out I am not really...that the ground I am "gaining" is only the result of how much I rest and the accommodations we make for my disease.

We keep thinking I am getting stronger and gaining more balance and coordination, and then we realize it is bullshit. It is striking to find out that you aren't getting stronger, even as you may be having moments of being more active and *feeling stronger*; that they are not moments of legitimately being stronger, just a result of being well-taken care of...of which I am so grateful!

I never want to sound ungrateful for how "pampered" I am, but it is upsetting to realize, yet again, that I am not actually any stronger than I may have been a couple of years ago. I just have the ability to rest so much more since Sage is more independent and not with me 24 hours a day, so I am not struggling so much with being worn out from keeping up with her. That means we see my *true disease* fatigue and lack of stamina come through. It highlights the constant and transitory need for rest and what it really does to keep me afloat.

It highlights two of the main problems with this dark disease. It shows that someone with one of these invisible, autoimmune, neuro-muscular (or similar) muscle diseases can be toolin' along, enjoying life, thinking they have a handle on their circumstance, and then BAM the disease puts a mountain in the road to remind you it is there and that it is still in charge.

It also, and this was possibly more startling and gutting, highlights how much of my independence is illusory. I am alone a lot, I do "things" alone. But when it comes down to it, I am so dependent on Scott (and others) for my safety and security. I am really not okay in this world alone. That may be the toughest pill to swallow of my entire medicine cabinet.

It seems, the reason I do so "well" is because I rest so much, I sleep half of most days while Scott works and Sage is gone at the rink and school, and when I do go places with Scott he takes such good care of me. When we go for walks, we hold hands, because we are so cheesy and just love to hold hands, even twenty years into our life together. But the truth is, he is so strong and aware of my movements, that he manages to steady me. It's not really because I am so much stronger. When we go for a leisurely bike ride, we map out the easiest ride for me with frequent stops. We bought me a comfort "city" bike with the easiest pedals, and Scott still has to sometimes retrieve me because I cannot finish.

What a harsh realization!

*When we get home from a walk (or bike ride), I sleep.

*When I go to the store alone, which is rare, I usually only go to one store at a time; and then I sit in the car to catch my breath before I drive and rest when I get home.

*When I go to the rink to watch Sage skate, I sit; and when I get to the car, I rest before I drive and rest when I get home.

*When I go to the doctor, I come home and go to bed.

*When I go with a friend to lunch or coffee, I *sit* and enjoy my friend, and then I come home and rest.

Every effort we make has a result, mine is sleep (or at least a heating pad, pillow, and lying down).

Falling made me realize I am not getting stronger. It encapsulates that I have just gotten better about managing my symptoms and accommodating for my weakness and lack of coordination with rest before and after activities; and have put systems into place to make those activities work for me.

In the end, though, I am still fighting this alone when I end up alone in my car trying to catch my breath. I am still alone inside my body, in bed, in pain after exertion. No amount of Scott rubbing my screaming muscles, or him holding me while I cry takes away the interior hell I am living. I am still the one falling for no apparent reason looking like a fucking idiot when no one else around me would fall — or at least be hurt if they fell — in that situation.

That sums up perfectly how my disease feels like a sentence of solitary confinement in the autoimmune abyss.

Chapter 14

Pain: What the Hell Is It and Who Gets to Determine If You Have It Anyway?

"You Don't Know About Me," by Ella Vos

Pain.

Myositis Pain.

All-over-body Pain.

Unrelenting, pull-your-hair-out, scream-at-the-top-of-your-lungs, cry-until-you-can't-see, Pain.

So-bad-you-can't-even-scream Pain.

You aren't making it up, and you aren't alone...Pain.

Until recently there was, what felt to many of us patients as, a heated debate, (or I will coin a new word: dis-consensus) among myositis "experts" about if myositis causes pain. In fact, I was at a conference once where a so-called "myositis expert" in one room denied there is pain in myositis as other "myositis experts" discussed the effects of myositis pain on patients in other rooms.

Doctors used to be taught lots of erroneous things that were harmful to patients. One was "If You Hear Hoof Beats, Think Horses, Not Zebras."[38] Another was that pain didn't occur in myositis (and is still being erroneously listed by some sources).[39] However most sources have been updated to include pain as a symptom.[40]

However, as patient groups became more active it was increasingly clear that those "experts" forgot to consult with the *real* Experts...the patients. Yes, we have pain. Yes, it is bad. Yes, it is widespread and diffuse. No, it is not only attributable to commingled fibromyalgia or other comorbidities. Yes, it is a clearly demarcated symptom that is 1) terrible and debilitating, 2) not in our heads, 3) clearly exacerbated during flares of myositis, 4) often becomes chronic, 5) in need of aggressive treatment to improve the quality of myositis patients' lives, and 6) doesn't always respond to pain medications the same way pain from an acute injury does.

Treating myositis patients, or other chronic illness patients for that matter, like criminals does nothing to honor the Hippocratic Oath. When I volunteered for MSU, one of the main complaints of our members was that doctors ignored pain. Often our patient-members would beg for relief and be told that the doctors' hands were tied due to the 2016 CDC opioid restrictions, however those guidelines were clearly written to state that people with chronic illnesses were not to be impacted. I have heard patients report that doctors would state that they could lose their licenses for giving them the pain meds they needed and doctors would taper their pain meds at such fast rates that patients would tell me, personally, they would rather die than live with the pain their doctors were forcing them to experience with such fast tapers.

I asked if they had told their doctors. Many told me the doctors responded their hands were tied, and if they needed more pain management, they had to go to the ER. However, if they went to the ER for more pain medication, they would be violating their "pain medication contracts." For some patients, to do so would result in being kicked out of that doctor's practice at least, and referral to criminal charges for misuse of controlled substances at worst. For a chronic illness patient, this is a scary, scary prospect. When we just want relief.

I am unable to take most opioids because of my stupid allergies, so I laugh at doctors and ER nurses when they accuse me of drug seeking, but it isn't as easy for many of my friends. Even though the CDC has clarified, multiple times, that the guidelines were not intended to hard people with chronic, intractable pain, doctors were just not listening.

In 2019, I helped formulate and administer an online survey of myositis patients about their pain, how their doctors were managing it, and if they were feeling the CDC guidelines, as reported by doctors, were infringing on their ability to get adequate pain coverage. In 2022, MSU's clinical advisors analyzed and had the significant results showing that myositis patients do indeed experience pain and that pain should be addressed as part of our treatment plans published in the medical journal, *Rheumatology*.[41] This is vindicating for patients who have been dismissed and belittled about their pain.

Since then, the CDC refined the guidelines again to emphasize that chronic illness patients with chronic pain were never intended to be caught up in the snare of the opioid crackdown.[42] The CDC acknowledges the harms caused by overzealous use of the 2016 guidelines in the 2022 reissued guidelines:

> Although some laws, regulations, and policies that appear to support recommendations in the 2016 CDC Opioid Prescribing Guideline might have had positive results for some patients, they are inconsistent with a central tenet of the guideline: that the recommendations are voluntary and intended to be flexible to support, not supplant, individualized, patient-centered care. Of particular concern,

some policies purportedly drawn from the 2016 CDC Opioid Prescribing Guideline have been notably inconsistent with it and have gone well beyond its clinical recommendations (6,66,67). Such misapplication includes extension to patient populations not covered in the 2016 CDC Opioid Prescribing Guideline (e.g., cancer and palliative care patients), rapid opioid tapers and abrupt discontinuation without collaboration with patients, rigid application of opioid dosage thresholds, application of the guideline's recommendations for opioid use for pain to medications for opioid use disorder treatment (previously referred to as medication assisted treatment), duration limits by insurers and pharmacies, and patient dismissal and abandonment (66–68). These actions are not consistent with the 2016 CDC Opioid Prescribing Guideline and have contributed to patient harm, including untreated and undertreated pain, serious withdrawal symptoms, worsening pain outcomes, psychological distress, overdose, and suicidal ideation and behavior (66–71).

Again, MSU is continuing to lead the charge to make sure that these egregious oversteps by doctors, relying on the 2016 guidelines to **cause harm to chronic illness and chronic pain patients** is stopped.

You probably notice that this chapter has a substantially different tone than all the others in this book...it is because I believe it is incumbent upon me to expose the darkness that is called "pain management."

I have had too many friends with myositis and with other types of *documented chronic pain* tell me that the chronic pain is so unbearable they would rather die. I know of at least one person who died by suicide due to the pain of myositis; and I suspect that there are others of my friends whose deaths were not accidental but were not publicly acknowledged as such.

I know from my own pain that there are times that the pain is so bad that if I did not have the resources I have for massage, acupuncture, and later access to legal cannabis to deaden the pain my nerve pain combined with my muscle contractions would breeder me inconsolable, and now that I have experienced the chemical suicidal ideations from medical side effects I know the spilt second decision it takes to end your life. Thankfully I did not do so, but in a moment of devastating physical pain compounded with emotional turmoil my story would — yes, I am saying **would** — have ended differently. These doctors are torturing patients by "following" guidelines.

Chapter 15

Sometimes I Need to Hold My Tongue or I'll End Up On TV:

How Love Keeps Me Going When I Want to Scream!

———

"'Til You're Home," from A Man called Otto by Rita Wilson and Sebastián Yatra

Right after I finished writing this book and had sent it off to a few people for review and editing I had an experience that couldn't be ignored so I'm inserting another chapter. That's the nature of autoimmune disease. These experiences keep happening. If I waited to stop writing, I'd never get this book out to you, dear reader.

Our 14-year-old dog, River, a yorkie (specifically an Australian Blue), had to have surgery on his luxating patella (aka an unstable kneecap). It had been planned for over a month. He has had intermittent trouble with his knee since he was a puppy, but it had always previously resolved on its own. In January 2023, it "went out" and he never stopped limping.

Aside from his own worth as a living being, which we take very seriously, and our dedication to his quality of life, River is my constant companion. He is always next to me for my infusions. When my head hurts, he curls himself around it. When I'm having a rough day, he is my living heating pad, and knows which part of my body to warm.

He is my protector (despite our "It's okay, mommy's got this" admonitions). He is very busy at his "job" and barks at all the dangerous birds, wind, and doorbells as well as any unknown person coming near me. Unfortunately, that means there are a couple of people who have experienced the sting of his bite as well as his bark. Fortunately, the people he has nipped are close to us and understand that he thinks he is my guard. This is how he has earned his accurate, and funny, online persona, "River 'the Asshole' Filmore" or "RTA." He enjoys posing for pictures and often asks me, "Why do people think I am an asshole when I am so cute and sweet, mama?" I'm waiting for the day there is a brain implant for dogs so I don't have to make up his voice and can hear it for real!

A pet taking on a caretaking role for a chronically ill person is a consistent experience across chronic illness people's stories.

I swear River is a person. He is my person, and I am his. He loves Sage and Scott. However, he thinks Scott is an interloper, and we often have to remind River that Scott is also *my person*; but he adores Scott too and the same in reverse. Just don't tell Scott I said so, he will deny it.

Anyway, back to River's surgery. When scheduling, I had asked all the questions I could think of about recovery and implications, indicating that I am disabled and have limited mobility, being the person who is home the most with River. The details were not spelled out prior to scheduling surgery in a way to indicate the severity of how much care he would need. We were told he needed the surgery. He would not be allowed to jump or climb the stairs and would need "rest" for 6-8 weeks. But not ever having had an animal have serious surgery like this, we didn't know what that entailed. We weren't given explicit instructions...until we picked him up.

We were told he couldn't do anything for himself at all for two weeks; and not much at all for eight. We were to keep him from running to the door to look outside. Keep him from jumping up and down from the couch. No standing on hind legs. No hopping, no stairs. No sudden movements. The list went on and on and on.

I started to panic. This dog may be fourteen, but he thinks he is *four*. I'm not kidding — he is faster, stronger, and lighter on his feet than any 14-year-old dog should be allowed to be (probably partly why his knee went out). ***And he is far stronger than me.***

As the vet stood in the lobby outlining all the restrictions to us, *post-op*, I started to panic and my thoughts started to race.

"I am home all day alone with this little fucker." (affectionately) "How the hell am I going to stop him if he suddenly tries to run off the couch? I can't just move that fast!" "What am I going to do to stop him from jumping? I can't stoop over and walk at the same time to pick him up! I have to tell him to sit, which he usually obeys, and then I can pick him up; but if he is not feeling well or in a bad mood or wanting to see something out the door, I won't be able to catch him! I just fell down the stairs ten days ago! I can't risk that again, how can I carry him up and down the stairs!?!?!?"

So, aloud, I said, "No one gave us an indication that he would be this restricted. I am disabled and he is stronger than me. I do not have the ability to contain him this much and I certainly cannot carry him up and down the stairs, every single time, for eight weeks."

She had the fucking audacity to look me up and down assessing me...you know what I'm talking about, the kind of withering look that chills you to your bones...and said in a haughty tone:

"How on earth is a 10-pound dog stronger than you?"

What the actual fuck? I just told this woman I am disabled. I get that I have an invisible disease, but she is a "medical professional" (albeit for animals) for crying out loud. Take a deep breath, Emily, River needs you, today is not the day to get arrested or be on the local news. DEEP BREATH...

Me: "Like I said, I have a muscle disease, and he is very much in fact stronger than me. I am very weak, with an invisible autoimmune disease. River on the other hand usually acts like a 4-year-old."

Her: flicking her hand at Scott and Sage: "Why can't **they** take care of him?"

[Okay bitty, now you questioned my disease **and** impugned my family.]

Me: "THEY ARE NOT AT HOME ALL DAY! I AM ALONE!"

Then she spouted some inhumane bullshit about leaving him, my poor baby who just had painful surgery which included the aforementioned luxating patella and an additional torn ligament, in crates all day and other crap that isn't happening because he is only part dog and mostly human with lots of hair. She offered to give us medications to keep him sedated along with lowering his pain (wow, how about offering that from the fucking start instead of questioning someone's disability???)

We got the hell out of there before I said something, hmmmmm, untoward.

Thankfully, Scott was able to work from home most of that initial week and we made a makeshift playpen out of the sectional sofa with our barstools to block River and me in. River and I slept most of that week, so that helped. Once he started doing better we had to restrict his movements by blocking pathways, but it worked out okay. Unfortunately, had we known the full extent of his recovery we would have planned the timing better. It was exhausting and taxing on my fragile body to add taking care of what amounted to a newborn baby who needed constant care.

Also, at the time we were getting ready to move, three weeks later, to a one-story home because I was having so much trouble with the stairs; packing, a dog who was recovering from knee surgery, and me struggling with this uncooperative body...these things didn't go well together.

The moral of this story? This is just an example of many other times I've had similar experiences of disdain and disbelief about my abilities and/or lack of abilities. I push through a lot of pain. I try to stand tall (figuratively). I try to be present with my family. I don't need the once over.

In the time since I wrote TMT, I've lost so many of the friends I've made through my connections at MSU and through my book due an extensive list of complications including bowel problems, heart and lung complications, blood clots, pneumonia, autoimmune-related cancer, falls, infections, aneurisms, medication side-effects, and even directly from their autoimmune disease or myositis complications. I don't take any day for granted and it continues to make me live as if I am dying.

Living fully for me looks a lot different than it does for a healthy person, and it includes hard crashes. It doesn't mean I am not in enormous amounts of pain; it doesn't mean my muscles aren't shaking and quaking. That doesn't mean that, while Scott and I are still very much in love and do enjoy hand holding and hugging, that many times I am also leaning on him for physical support. If you were to see me at one of Sage's skating competitions, I am almost always leaning, sitting, or finding a quiet area to rest in between the times I am "on" for Sage.

This is how it is for so many of my friends, they do what they do to be part of their family and then they suffer the consequences later. We sleep for days after an event or holiday. We take on extra pain for a few hours of being part of our kids' lives. We take a lot of extra pain meds, smoke some extra weed, take some emergency doses of the dreaded steroids, and then sleep — sleep — sleep to recover.

But that isn't without limits. Scott protects me. He "babies" and "caretakes" me in a kind and loving way that is not demeaning, is respectful, but has enriched and likely lengthened my life immensely. I don't know how I would ever thank him or repay him enough, so I just love him and our kids the best I can. That's all I can do — and when someone is a complete and utter asshole like the vet I mentioned above, I try not to make an ass out of myself so as not to embarrass him **too much**.

But I guess the real answer to these situations is to try to ask more questions. Press for more information **beforehand**. Make people explain everything! Trust no one to give you information freely.

You would think that I would know this after nearly three decades of surviving this bullshit. But I clearly still need to work at my own pre-communication with others. I still must work to be okay enough with myself to live with the ignorant disdain of others over an illness I can't control. I still need to remember that it is okay to get my feelings hurt and it is acceptable to get angry when someone treats me inappropriately.

I know I am not alone in these experiences. I have never been confronted directly about my disabled parking placard, but I have seen the sneers and heard mutterings under peoples' breath. I have friends who have been questioned by "concerned parties."

My friend Angi who lives with another chronic condition said this, "Almost everyone can say they have been 'looked at' that way where they felt they had to defend themselves and explain the 'whys.' **Why** do you have a parking placard, when you don't look disabled? **Why** do you need pain meds? You must be a drug seeker, you are not sick enough to need them! **Why** can't you: work, go out with us, come over for a while to watch my kids, take care of the little dog on your own? You went out last week! **Why** are you pretending you can't get up the steps, you don't look like anything's wrong with your legs? The list of 'whys' is endless."

The thing that people who ask questions like what I faced, what you may face, and what my friend Angi is talking about is that with dynamic, cyclical, and chronic conditions is we don't know from hour-to-hour, day-to-day, much less week-to-week what we will be able to do. It is complete hog wash to judge our existence or actions based on something we attempted to do a week ago. The person asking probably has no clue the amount of rest, pain, and medication it took to make up for that exertion. Sometimes I wish I was way less polite than I am, and could just say, aloud, "butt the fuck out." Because *you know* I'm saying it in my head!

Invisible diseases are real. They are no less life changing than visible ones. We exist. We suffer. We deserve compassion. We **need** our accommodations to survive much less thrive (and yes, we do deserve to do more than survive). We have the right to be in the world without disdain and without being questioned and interrogated. *We don't owe anyone an explanation.*

Because goddamnit...being sick sucks enough without other people making it worse.

Chapter 16
What Does Stronger Mean, Anyway?

———

"Stronger (What Doesn't Kill You)," by Kelly Clarkson

and

"Roar," by Katy Perry

The whole time I have been writing this book, Connie has been asking me, is writing it cathartic? You know, she wants to know if the act of vomiting my feelings onto the page helping me! It has, it is kind of like an ongoing therapy session within myself. I think it is cathartic, but it is also motivating.

Am I healthier than I was when I started writing? Well, I am not still paranoid from the increased pulse of steroids, so check! I am no longer suicidal from the jak inhibitor, so check! I think as we know about journaling, drawing, music, and all the creative endeavors, getting your feelings out helps, so I do think writing this has helped me. I feel buoyed by the idea that I may help a few people with my writing. I also resumed acupuncture since I started writing, which has helped with my stress levels, my pain, and other small and transitory changes that would be too hard to pinpoint.

Am I physically better, overall? No, my disease is refractory and cyclical. I continue to have ups and downs.

Does that matter at this point? Maybe not.

Maybe writing it has brought me back to a place of reality and acceptance. I think I had started to believe my circumstance was changing. (It is. I can, in fact, walk a little better than I could 2-3 years ago.) I started to have cognitive dissonance (holding two contrary beliefs about myself)[43] again

But I would like to leave you with some ideas of things we can do to better our day when the shit just seems to keep coming like a monkey throwing its poop at you.

A few years ago, a friend posted this story on Facebook encouraging you to run the dishwasher twice. Rather than feel guilty about being too tired to rinse the dishes "correctly," rerun it! If you do not dry the laundry fast enough before it mildews, just rerun it! Live without guilt over the things you cannot control.

Talk to an empathetic friend who will listen and not try to problem solve for you. Ask them beforehand if they are willing and able to do so, first!

Volunteer for a Patient-led organization related to your condition. Many of them allow you to do small tasks from home that don't take much time. Doing so helps you to feel needed and can clear out those cobwebs from the brain!

Listen to music. Even if you are stuck in bed, music is a nice way to soothe yourself, to feel connected to the world, and to find enjoyment.

Journal your feelings. Writing them down is powerful. You basically read excerpts from a short time of the journal of my life. It doesn't have to be formal...a few words a day work!

Get some crayons or colored pencils and color or do a paint by number. I have a friend who paints, in bed(!) every day! They say it brings them great joy!

If you don't have enough hand mobility for things like these, watch travel shows and explore the world from your bedroom!

Eat something decadent occasionally. Of course, healthy food is important to feed our bodies, but so is moderation and enjoyment!

If you can get outside, go for a short walk or a roll. Take a drive if possible. Find a way to see nature or use your computer to go to nature photo sites and look at the majesty of nature!

Read a book! Find something you love to do and do it!

And...Let it out! Scream. Cry. Yell into your pillow.

Consider taking a break from reading to listen to *"Let it Go," by Idina Menzel, from Frozen* (sing along at the loudest your energy and voice will allow if moved to do so!).

Know that there is no right or wrong way to cope with the feelings these horrible diseases thrust upon us, as long as you do it safely and are not harming yourself or others. I think, looking back over this book, you can almost see my attitude change.

The end of the book feels just a little less angry, maybe slightly less hopeless, even though I fell on my ass and I had a breakdown over understanding that this is here to stay. I still came to understand that it is okay to be pissed and upset; I had forgotten that, and I think in pushing those feelings down I had started to become bitter instead of following my own advice of letting feelings flow through me. That's largely part of telling my story. Getting it out — on to the page — in my case is cathartic, just as Connie thought,

Remember: Your feelings matter, you matter, and it is okay to *not be okay* because, Being Sick Sucks. You don't have to be alone staring into the autoimmune abyss, I am here. Others are also here. There are many support groups. If you have myositis check out Myositis Support and Understanding.

You can contact me through Facebook.

With infinite peace and love,

Emily <3

PS. When you close this book, both your new journey and the abyss await, hopefully slightly transformed. Until you are ready to read my other book, *The Marvelous Transformation,* I would love for you to listen to *"Unwritten," by Natasha Bedingfield.*

Acknowledgments

I stopped writing for a few years. I was content to bloviate on Facebook, document my health on Facebook in hopes of helping de-mystify myositis and autoimmune disease to my small friends list, write some articles for MSU (which I also eventually stopped), antagonize politicians on Twitter, and send angry (many) or supportive (some) letters to my representatives asking for change and exalting their good works in the plight of marginalized persons and human rights overall. Writing became too hard. I was having so much trouble with my eyes, I was tired of being sick while pretending — even to those closest to me that I was handling it okay, and the COVID pandemic took a toll on me. Far before that, I realized that I was expending too much of my limited energy, even at only 15 minutes per day, writing and then trying to figure out how to market my books. I started to think it didn't matter anyway. Nothing was going to change, we all kept getting sicker, the healthcare system didn't change, the medications didn't get better, the ones they have didn't really make me better, just helped me tread water, and my community seemed to be at a standstill. So I think I partially threw in the towel on making it better.

I was weary, drained, and not being a good mom. So, I walked away. I have a finite amount of energy. I have a finite amount of emotional currency. I have a finite amount of life. I decided to sink that back into my family.

The community and camaraderie I had built over the years with people living with myositis and autoimmune diseases and other chronic illnesses stayed, thankfully. I had come to rely on them for comfort, and for some reason, in turn, many people had come to count on me for comfort and information. That was enough for me.

Then some of my people helped me find the courage to write this book and use this part of my story to help others, somehow, someway, within my limitations. Even if it meant dictating it sentence by sentence into my phone to edit later (which I did sometimes). Other people gave me encouragement, others gave me space to grieve my illness, and still others helped us ensure Sage was safe which freed up my body, mind, and soul to even attempt to write again. These are their stories.

*By the way, I have countless people in my life who I could write about here for the ways in which they have helped on this autoimmune journey. This time, I am going to limit it to those who directly impacted the book. But please know, I am thinking of every single one of you who has helped me throughout the years.

Connie when you asked, well, I think you demanded, that I write this book, I had been having the itch, but not the energy, to write. Without your prodding and encouragement, this book would not exist. So, readers, if you hate it, blame her. If you love it, well, I am the author so it's all me! Ha Ha, just kidding...She gets at least half the credit. Thank you, Connie for your support, your encouragement, and believing I could do it all over again. You are a gift!

Mara, we survived the pandemic by social distancing in the driveway, then on the front porch. I guess the saying is right that pressure produces strength, because you and I came out of it stronger friends than ever! Thank you for being my friend and helping me through some of the toughest times through now. You are a continued rock I can lean on, and hope I am the same for you.

Coach Chris, having spent most of Sage's life with her within constant arms' reach, it was hard for me to let her fly. As she grows up it is important to me to know she is safely ensconced in a positive environment for her next steps. Your love for humanity, the way you see the world, and the way that you empathize with the plight of others makes the decision Scott and I made to move here so you could coach her so much better. We are happy that you are helping us usher her into the next phase of her life. Your coaching and just being you, knowing that you have her back, has brightened our lives tremendously and gave me the peace to be able to write this book. Thank you.

On that note, Lauren, your contributions in helping Sage traverse life with a sick mom are priceless and make our entire life better. Thank you!

Robyn, thank you for listening without judgment when I have one of the no-good, horrible, rotten days described here. You have quickly become someone invaluable in my and Sage's life, and I hope we can continue to build our beautiful friendship in the coming years.

Jerry and Sandy, we started MSU together and although our lives have slightly diverged since, this book would not be possible without your love, the lessons I learned, and the beautifully important and powerful thing we built. I am forever grateful for our friendship, proud of what we made, and that it continues to thrive with the current team; especially Lynn, who I dearly thank for her leadership and friendship.

Amy, you have always been there for me since the day we met under the "Columns" at Westminster. I am not sure who, or where, I would be without you, your love, support, and honesty. You taught me what it meant to be accepted for who I am. You are like one of my limbs. Thank you for always being there to lend your open heart to me. I love and cherish you.

Angi, I am grateful for you and our decades of friendship. You have an uncanny way of sending me notes when I need them. You don't seem to realize it, but you have an infectious and joyous way about you that encourages and buoys the people you care about. You are giving and loving, and I am so grateful to be a recipient of your light.

Your encouragement about my writing and why it is important to do this helped me keep going when "I don't wanna write anymore." Your patience also helps me when I don't have any patience left with my own body. I love and thank you.

Jaime, you continue to save me from myself (and commas) every day. Thank you for editing this book for me and for making sure I look and sound good (well? Shit, you better fix that!)! You know (as we keep telling Sage while she traverses the trials and tribulations of emerging into adulthood) that I would not be who I am if we didn't take that fateful road trip to clear our minds in the fall of '95 and you opened my mind to a different perspective than I had experienced before. We entered that car suitemates and left it knowing we were soulmates. You not only edit my writing, but you keep me grounded, you challenge me to think outside of my experience, and you taught me the value of caring more about another person than myself. We've shared every secret, every heartbreak, every joy, and every growth moment imaginable in this life. You've saved my life more times than I care to acknowledge, most recently was literally spending four hours on the phone talking to me and keeping me safe while the medicine that tried to kill me wore off. You are the best. I hope I am half as good a friend to you as you are to me. In the immortal words of Kelly Clarkson, "My life would suck without you!"

Ty, you brighten my dark days. Thank you for always checking on me when your mom and I are on the phone. You are a special, dynamic, and amazing young man. Your contribution to the book was my worrying about being banished to outer space, or a cussing chair. I thought long and hard about it, but I have instead, included an article for you to read on the honesty of people who cuss! I love you.[44]

Drew, Lucas, and Colin, even though we don't live in the same city anymore, your presence is still felt deeply in my life. I love watching the kids flourish and Drew, your calls with stories and silly antics still bring me so much laughter and fun in what can be a boring and lonely day. Your visits during the pandemic were crucial to our ability to stay safe and happy and we cannot ever convey to you what they meant to us.

Dad and Marti, this long and winding road has brought us to a place that I love in our relationship. I know I get my writing talent from you, Dad, so there is your credit! I appreciate all you have done to help me along the way as I have battled these awful circumstances. I got my tenacity, my sense of standing strong in my beliefs, and if anyone thinks I have a temper, which I don't, my temper all came from you. We don't always agree, but I'm glad we are finally old enough to realize it doesn't matter. I love you.

Rickey and Tiffany, my grown-up loves. You continue to amaze me with your love for the world, your love for each other, your love for our family, and each of your passions for your chosen life's work. Anytime I ask, "do you think I can do this?" Your answer is always, "Do it safely, but try it!" and when my body fails me you never express disappointment, you never say "it sucks," you just thank me for being here, safe, thank me for trying (for **me** not you), and for being okay. When I succeed you are the biggest cheerleaders right along with Scott and Sage. I don't know how much more supportive kids could be of an ill parent but to accept the truth, and also be there with me as I try to increase my stability or strength or stamina, sometimes succeeding and sometimes falling short. During the pandemic you helped keep me safe beyond anything we could have imagined. I'm sorry for the sucky parts but I'm really glad you are with me. This book wouldn't exist without you in so many ways, especially your encouragement and love. I love you more.

Sagey-poo, you have been through hell. I wish I could have saved you from how much it sucks to have a sick mommy. It isn't fair, but you have grown into an intelligent, independent, well-spoken, empathetic, and witty young woman who can take on this world with a wealth of experience, knowledge, and joy behind and in front of you. I am proud to be your mama and I thank you for putting up with all the meds, needles, infusions, doctor visits, hospitals, falls, crying, smells, scary wake-ups, and all the other things that went bump in the night or day that I can never make up for but know happened and affected you deeply. I hope someday, you will forgive me and the universe and find your own bright side, because you, my sweet, sweet darling shine brighter than any star in the galaxy. You deserve happiness and will have it. Daddy and I will be right here to catch you when you need us and will be here to smile, applaud, and cheer for you when you don't.

To my ultimate protector, my shadow, my partner-in-crime, my very favorite "person" — River (the Asshole) Filmore. Thank you for always being there for me, even when I don't want you to be. *If you don't already know, River is my dog and is the bestest and worstest behaved boy in the world who loves me more than anyone!

Scott, my beloved. We both know DM would have destroyed me by now if it weren't for you. How do you thank the person who holds you up when you don't think you have anything left to stand with? How do you acknowledge the person who believes in you when you don't? It's impossible. I try to tell you, privately, loudly, publicly, any way possible, daily and in million ways. But I'll just say it again. Thank you for being my #1. Thank you for putting up with my illnesses and taking care of me, for pretending to enjoy my jokes, and for always catching me when I fall (if you are there). I hope I am half the partner to you as you are to me. I **love** and **cherish** and **like** you.

Notations

Notes, Endnotes, and Citations

[1] https://www.dictionary.com/browse/abyss

[2] Nietzsche can be a controversial philosophical figure. History isn't exactly sure of what to make of him, so I struggled with the decision to put his quote here because I do not condone hatred, past or present. However, contrary to co-opting by certain modern hate groups, multiple accounts emphasize that he was against antisemitism, and his message was manipulated to look different later.

[3] Daniel Howell's quote is from this video where he talks about his thoughts on existentialism. He is a person just like you and me, but I love his quote as it relates to my journey with autoimmune disease: https://www.youtube.com/watch?v=B1jaY136B_k

[4] https://ccprcentre.org/ccpr-board-staff

[5] https://www.apa.org/monitor/mar01/synesthesia

[6] Filmore, Emily. *The Marvelous Transformation*. Central Recovery Press, LLC, 22 June 2015.

[7] https://www.britannica.com/science/hoarfrost

[8] Poe, Edgar Allan, Symons, Julian. **The Tell-Tale Heart: The Life and Works of Edgar Allan Poe.** Dallas: Penguin Books, 1978.

[9] https://www.gsb.stanford.edu/faculty-research/publications/frankly-we-do-give-damn-relationship-between-profanity-honesty

[10] Please note: this book is happening in real time. I write in the moment and this disease is ever-changing and ever evolving. Even as I go back and edit sometimes things have changed and I will note them too. Timelines don't necessarily matter for our purposes, but if they do, I will do my best to notate chronological order; but mostly I'll let the story flow and evolve as my life and disease does, because that's how

the Autoimmune abyss works, isn't it? The only two ways to prevent that would be 1) to write it in one sitting – which is not going to happen! 2) to try to confine the book into a neat little outline and not deviate. My brain doesn't work like that and I think it would stunt the book and block the flow of ideas; making it less **real.**

[11] List of my books:

Filmore, Emily A. *It's a Beautiful Day for Yoga.* Beautiful Day Publishing, 2009.

Filmore, Emily A. *It's a Beautiful Day for a Walk.* Beautiful Day Publishing, 2010.

Walsch, Neale Donald, et al. *Conversations with God for Parents: Sharing the Messages with Children.* Square One Publishing, 2017.

Farley, Laurie Lankins, & Filmore, Emily A. *Parenting through Divinity.* Waterside Productions, 2018.

[12] **Wachowski, L., & Wachowski, L. (1999).** The Matrix. Warner Bros.

[13] https://www.sciencedaily.com/releases/2011/08/110824122906.htm

[14]   https://www.propublica.org/article/unitedhealth-healthcare-insurance-denial-ulcerative-colitis?fbclid=IwAR36aJQs_u_dzQk69CL1Nj-U8t8kWgcCRgl6d8K61iY4vb4O0774E6JFY48&mibextid=ykz3hl

[15]   https://cptsdfoundation.org/what-is-complex-post-traumatic-stress-disorder-cptsd/

[16]   https://themighty.com/topic/chronic-illness/chronic-illness-induced-ptsd-trauma/

[17]   https://www.instagram.com/p/Cn-u7LpM_7t/?igshid=NTU1Mzc3ZGM%3D&fbclid=IwAR3ltw-SPnhJj3sxy3EPfCSnfdxK42-_NCs51-3OuFcvgaQ-fp57QVHPUZw[1]

[18] Garfunkel, introducing the song at a live performance (with Simon) in Harlem, June 1966, summed up the song's meaning as "the inability of people to communicate

---

1. https://www.instagram.com/p/Cn-u7LpM_7t/?igshid=NTU1Mzc3ZGM=&fbclid=IwAR3ltw-SPnhJj3sxy3EPfCSnfdxK42-_NCs51-3OuFcvgaQ-fp57QVHPUZw

with each other, not particularly intentionally but especially emotionally, so what you see around you are people unable to love each other."

Retrieved on 12/19/2022 from https://en.wikipedia.org/wiki/The_Sound_of_Silence#cite_ref-Eliot40_11-1 referencing https://archive.org/details/paulsimonlife0000elio/page/40/mode/2up

[19] https://themighty.com/topic/rare-disease/rare-disease-advocacy-emergency-room/?fbclid=IwAR1SfCNX_mj3_-o0QVvLaGCq5Tth-F7nzYzhhi3MRmJHpOoIO6pphqNjbj8_aem_AUVvIhv-QoJ_M7p-xsnMDRu9iNBttsjIZu3SqzvzMaVlYGaGN2vIDWnTgmj8Ys77_Wc

[20] https://www.ncbi.nlm.nih.gov/pmc/articles/PMC4354806/

[21] https://www.healthline.com/health-news/this-med-student-wrote-the-book-on-diagnosing-disease-on-darker-skin

[22] https://www.medpagetoday.com/opinion/second-opinions/97383

[23] https://understandingmyositis.org/myositis/dermatomyositis/ and https://rarediseases.org/rare-diseases/dermatomyositis/

[24] See Article 25. https://www.un.org/sites/un2.un.org/files/2021/03/udhr.pdf

[25] https://www.ncbi.nlm.nih.gov/books/NBK459441/

[26] https://understandingmyositis.org/myositis-complications/myositis-cancer/

[27] https://www.refinery29.com/en-gb/what-are-dynamic-disabilities

[28] Kendi, I.X. (2019). How to be an Antiracist. Random House Publishing Group. and Fleming, Heather S. (2019). My Black Friend Says…: Lessons in Equity, Inclusion, and Cultural Competency.

[29] https://www.healthline.com/health-news/this-med-student-wrote-the-book-on-diagnosing-disease-on-darker-skin

[30] https://www.merriam-webster.com/dictionary/altruism

[31] https://www.hrw.org/report/2022/04/12/if-im-out-insulin-im-going-die/united-states-lack-regulation-fuels-crisis

32   https://www.billboard.com/music/pop/alessia-cara-hair-loss-scars-to-your-beautiful-7468466/

33 Perry, Matthew. *Friends, Lovers, and the Big Terrible Thing: A Memoir*. New York, NY: Flatiron Books, 2022.

34 "Addiction is a lot like other diseases, such as heart disease. Both disrupt the normal, healthy functioning of an organ in the body, both have serious harmful effects, and both are, in many cases, preventable and treatable. If left untreated, they can last a lifetime and may lead to death." https://nida.nih.gov/publications/drugs-brains-behavior-science-addiction/drug-misuse-addiction

35 "Mental illness is nothing to be ashamed of. It is a medical problem, just like heart disease or diabetes." https://www.psychiatry.org/patients-families/what-is-mental-illness

36 Perry, Matthew. *Friends, Lovers, and the Big Terrible Thing: A Memoir*. New York, NY: Flatiron Books, 2022. Pg. 202.

37 Some suicide hotlines and other information:

In the US is: 988 or https://988lifeline.org.

In the UK: 0800 689 5652 or https://www.spuk.org.uk/national-suicide-prevention-helpline-uk/

In Canada: 211 or https://211lifeline.org/detail.php?id=53773170

In South Africa: https://www.gov.za/world-suicide-prevention-day

The World Health Organization (WHO) is working to prevent suicide in Africa as a whole, more information can be found here: https://www.afro.who.int/news/reversing-suicide-mental-health-crisis-africa

Here is a page with a more worldwide listing: https://america.cgtn.com/2015/03/05/find-help-for-suicide-prevention-centers-around-the-world

*You can always call your doctor or emergency medical services (911 in the US), as well as a trusted family member.

38 https://www.ncbi.nlm.nih.gov/pmc/articles/PMC5072891/

[39] https://www.mountsinai.org/care/rheumatology/services/myositis Retrieved on 4/17/2023 "Myositis is an inflammatory condition that affects the muscles. There are several types of myositis, most of which are highly treatable. Symptoms of myositis typically involve weakness such a having trouble standing up from a chair, climbing stairs, lifting the arms. *But usually there is no muscle pain.* The weakness is typically symmetrical; it affects both legs or both arms, not just one." [Emphasis added]

[40] https://www.ncbi.nlm.nih.gov/pmc/articles/PMC5857275/

[41]   https://www.ncbi.nlm.nih.gov/pmc/articles/PMC9788817/   & https://academic.oup.com/rheumatology/article/62/1/264/6586791

[42]https://www.cdc.gov/mmwr/volumes/71/rr/ rr7103a1.htm?fbclid=IwAR1lgocNYwrARdWTICcmIsUChDvqgxOoTdficTXrvVuvDN0crjx_N (retrieved April 18, 2023)

[43] https://www.medicalnewstoday.com/articles/326738

[44] https://www.gsb.stanford.edu/faculty-research/publications/frankly-we-do-give-damn-relationship-between-profanity-honesty

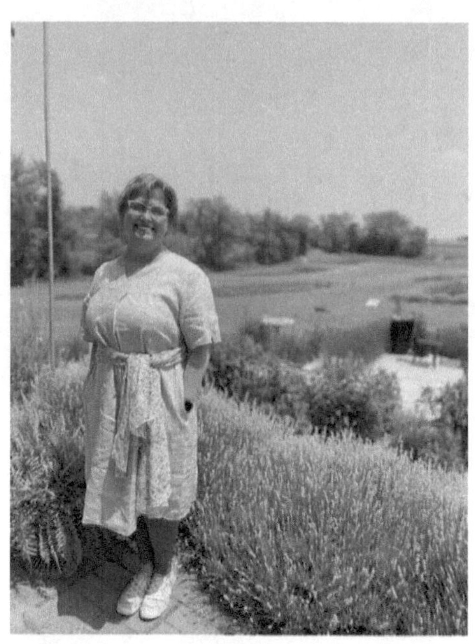

About the Author

Emily lives in Minnesota where she and Scott have discovered they actually really like Minnesota's winters! She cannot believe Sage and Rickey are all "grown up," River is still her annoying companion, and that her dermatomyositis won't go away!

Emily has a BA in Psychology and a Juris Doctor, but because of her autoimmune disease they are mostly good for arguing politics and human rights online, oh, and writing books.

When she isn't housebound in pain, she loves going for walks in the fresh Minnesota air with her cute hubby, looking at the beautiful flowers in her garden, drinking coffee on her deck, fighting with the chipmunk in her garden that hates her, and talking to friends and loved ones online and on the phone. She is a voracious reader and has already read over 65 books in 2023. Her kids and her husband are her love and joy.

Emily is the author of *The Marvelous Transformation: Living Well with Autoimmune* Disease (Central Recovery Press, 2015). She is also the co-author of *Conversations with God for Parents* with Neale Donald Walsch and Laurie Lankins Farley (Rainbow Ridge, 2015), *Parenting through Divinity* with Laurie Lankins Farley (Waterside Productions, 2018), and is sole author of the *With My Child Series* of children's books: *It's a Beautiful Day for Yoga* and *It's a Beautiful Day for a Walk* (Beautiful Day Publishing, 2009 and 2010, respectively).

Read more at https://www.facebook.com/emilyfilmoreauthor.